The Hidden Among the Hidden

The Hidden Among the Hidden

African-American Elder Male Caregivers

Helen K. Black
John T. Groce
and
Charles E. Harmon

OXFORD
UNIVERSITY PRESS

OXFORD
UNIVERSITY PRESS

Oxford University Press is a department of the University of Oxford. It furthers the University's objective of excellence in research, scholarship, and education by publishing worldwide. Oxford is a registered trade mark of Oxford University Press in the UK and certain other countries.

Published in the United States of America by Oxford University Press
198 Madison Avenue, New York, NY 10016, United States of America.

Library of Congress Cataloging-in-Publication Data
Names: Black, Helen K., 1952– author. | Groce, John T., 1932– author. | Harmon, Charles E., 1931– author.
Title: The hidden among the hidden : African-American elder male caregivers / by Helen K. Black, John T. Groce, and Charles E. Harmon.
Description: Cambridge ; New York, NY : Oxford University Press, [2017] | Includes bibliographical references and index.
Identifiers: LCCN 2016047455 (print) | LCCN 2017004453 (ebook) | ISBN 9780190602321 (alk. paper) | ISBN 9780190602338
Subjects: LCSH: Older African Americans—Family relationships. | African American men—Family relationships. | African American caregivers. | African American families.
Classification: LCC E185.86 .B5235 2017 (print) | LCC E185.86 (ebook) | DDC 306.85/08996073—dc23
LC record available at https://lccn.loc.gov/2016047455

1 3 5 7 9 8 6 4 2

Printed by Sheridan Books, Inc., United States of America

This book is dedicated
in loving memory of

Helen A. Black and Patricia Black Hrusko
(H. K. Black)

and

Rosetta Anderson Groce
You will always be the wind beneath my wings
(John T. Groce)

It is also dedicated to:

Constance Stevens Harmon
Who continues to keep me strong
(Charles E. Harmon)

ACKNOWLEDGMENTS

The authors are especially grateful to the men who allowed us to interview them. With warmth, courage, and candor, they shared with us the stories of giving care to their loved ones. Because there are so few narratives of care told by African-American men, we acknowledge them as the forerunners they are as caregivers and as men.

The authors also wish to thank the following individuals: Louis Colbert, who wrote the foreword for this book; Christa Caruso for transcribing the interviews; Robert L. Rubinstein, who read drafts of the manuscript and offered comments and guidance; and Jeninne Groce Martin, who provided us with a comprehensive list of resources to assist caregivers. We extend our gratitude to our family members and dear friends who encouraged us in this endeavor and anticipated its publication.

We also thank the editors and anonymous reviewers from Oxford University Press who accepted our manuscript and offered advice, critiques, and suggestions regarding its content.

CONTENTS

FOREWORD

I grew up in a family with six siblings, my father, mother, and maternal grandmother. The grown-ups molded the foundation that shaped our character. My first caregiving experience happened the summer after seventh grade. My grandmother suffered from phlebitis, which caused swelling in her legs. The treatment required that her legs be elevated most of the day. So my job that summer was to answer her bell when she rang, at any time, for anything she needed. My job was to attend to her every need. It never crossed my mind I was a caregiver because it seldom kept me off the baseball diamond or out of a good game of hide-and-seek. It was what we knew because it mirrored our whole lives.

My father was a healthy, tall, lean man. I never knew him to be sick. He was a letter carrier who walked his route for over 30 years. Retirement was good. In the summer of 2003, I remember him making a remark about a pain in his side that he would attend to after he took care of Helen's (his wife, our mother) "honey do list." Helen's honey do list was finished in late November, and he finally went to the doctor. He learned he had pancreatic cancer and died on his birthday in February. It was quick, with very little suffering.

After my father died, my mother's health declined. It was gradual and lengthy. She suffered with heart disease, Parkinson's, diabetes, and dementia. Over the course of a year she went from being an independent decision maker who still drove to a woman who could barely walk and had a hospital bed and commode in the dining room. As the decline continued, she entered the PACE program, which allowed us to keep her at home and out of an institution. During her last 5 years, between siblings and her grandchildren, she was never left alone. As her needs grew greater, the caregiving demands grew heavier.

As an African-American male caregiver, I wish this book had been written 10 years ago. I am a trained geriatric social worker with over 38 years of experience in the field. I also facilitate a monthly caregiver support group at my church. But when I had to step up to the caregiver plate, I felt so unprepared, so frightened, so alone, and so confused as to where to turn for help on this journey. I repeat: I wish this book had been written 10 years ago.

The authors are caregivers and provided care collectively for over 40 years. This book shares the stories of 13 men—men we see in our barber shops, our churches, our drug stores, and on the job. They are policemen, teachers, plumbers, butchers, and bakers—all who have traveled this journey called caregiving. We know that 40% of all caregiving is done by men, and yet almost no research exists on older African-American males as informal caregivers. This book presents an in-depth portrait of caregivers who are considered "the hidden among the hidden."

The book is important because the authors successfully challenge two critical myths about African-American men. First, African-American men *do* care for other people. A recurring theme in the narratives of spousal caregivers is that the men stayed married for a long, long time. The second myth addressed by the authors is about the nurturing ability of African-American men. It is critical that the perceptions of African-American men be shifted to men who remain long married, become caregivers, and remain committed to their families and communities throughout their lives. This book successfully does just that.

This is an invaluable, extraordinary book written with clarity, depth, and candor. The authors attempt to bring a more balanced depiction of African-American strengths in the face of oppression that marked the daily lives of their respondents. Birthed after the Million Man March, this book appears at a time when so many boomers are sandwiched between older and younger generations of loved ones, all of whom need their care. The number of African-American older adults who will need some manner of care is expected to triple by the year 2030, and this book can help families confront the coming caregiving tsunami. This book is not just for men, not just for African Americans, and not just for caregivers or care recipients. It is for everyone because we foresee that at some point most of us will be caregivers. And with this book you will be, unlike me, better prepared to face this tremendous journey of caregiving. The journey of 13 men is poignant, powerful, and fulfilling. "Each narrative includes accounts of the past, as well as the present, and shows the continuity of the respondent's life through time. Even after the care recipient's death, the caregiver continued to interpret the caregiving experience as meaningful" (see Chapter One, p. 13).

The book examines aspects of the caregiving experience and suggests that such qualities as patience, courage, trust, humility, knowledge, and hope are combined in the African-American caregiver package, which these men have demonstrated so well. For several of the men, including me, the caregiving experience is (or was) the last physical act of love that we are (or were) able to give our loved one.

As more men continue to provide care for loved ones, this book will help us look at African-American male caregivers from a fresh perspective. The authors successfully enlighten the world that there are many sides to every caregiver.

I salute the authors for this courageous story that had to be told. I know you will enjoy this book as much as I.

Be well.

Louis G. Colbert, MSW
Vice President of Operations
Philadelphia Corporation for Aging
Philadelphia, PA

PREFACE

WHAT THIS BOOK IS ABOUT

This book is about African-American elder male caregivers. Its title, *The Hidden Among the Hidden*, provides a clue about the need for such a book. Although statistics differ according to the source cited, families of all ethnicities are said to provide 90% of all home care for elderly relatives who are cognitively or physically impaired or both. Most caregivers are women, and nearly one in ten caregivers is over 75 years of age (National Caregiving Alliance [NAC] and the American Association of Retired Persons [AARP], 2015).

The picture of an informal caregiver, or one who is unpaid and is usually a family member, is that of a woman, often a daughter, daughter-in-law, or wife (NAC and AARP, 2015). Yet current estimates show that men make up nearly 40% of unpaid family care and have been dubbed "hidden caregivers" (Kramer & Thompson, 2005; NCA & AARP, 2015). Although we are not certain how many male caregivers of all ethnicities are elders (over 60), most sources suggest that the number of elder male caregivers providing hands-on care to loved ones, particularly spouses, is growing (NCA & AARP, 2015; Pharr, Francis, Terry, & Clark, 2014).

There is little research and literature on elder men as caregivers of demented or disabled loved ones (Black, Schwartz, Caruso, & Hannum, 2008; Kramer & Thompson, 2005). This may be due to the fact that there are fewer men than women caregivers, and that men may be reluctant or unable to join a focus group or be part of a survey on this topic, which are two major ways of collecting data on caregivers and caregiving. What is known about male caregivers agrees on four major points: They are likely to (1) feel unprepared for caregiving; (2) hesitate to request formal and informal assistance; (3) be unaware of resources that could aid them; and (4) be reluctant to talk about caregiving (Kramer & Thompson, 2005).

The aforementioned points regarding men's hiddenness in caregiving—from a sense of unpreparedness, continued through unawareness of resources, to a reluctance to discuss caregiving or requesting help—may come from several sources. One is a man's perception that he is not a caregiver, but rather "a needed husband doing what needed to be done" (see Chapter Two: case of Mr. Parker). Women are seen as "natural" caregivers because assisting those in distress traditionally has been viewed as "feminine" qualities (Kleinhman, 1980; Martin, 1987). Likewise, men's hesitancy to converse about their needs as caregivers may be part of the cultural construction of masculinities, or notions about how men 'should' behave when faced with caregiving (Lin, Fee, & Wu, 2012). For example, men's perceived appropriate reaction when faced with hardship may be to remain silent and stoic, which is an aspect of Western cultural and social legacies about gender-appropriate behavior (Lotterhos, 2015). Added to men's silence about caregiving is their apprehension about whether they are performing the role well or even adequately, which speaks to men's unease about their competency in caregiving and reluctance to share this concern (Black et al., 2008; Lin et al., 2012).

Because of the paucity of research on older male caregivers in general and particularly older African-American caregivers, we are uncertain whether African-American men have concerns about caregiving that are similar to other groups. Although African Americans in general are less likely to use formal support services (Lin et al., 2012; Pharr et al., 2014), they will turn to other family members, friends, neighbors, and fellow church members for informal support (Mattis et al., 2001). As we will learn from our caregiving respondents, however, giving physical and emotional care to others is an aspect of African Americans' inheritance from their distant and recent past (Pharr et al., 2014).

OUR PREMISE

Thus, the premise of this book is that caregiving is intricately and complexly tied to being an African American, to the community-oriented culture of African Americans, and to having experienced a history of exclusion and segregation (Black & Rubinstein, 2001; David, 2013; Mutua, 2006; Pharr et al., 2014). That is, experiences of racism and caregiving are intertwined; they are intensely and fiercely embedded in African-American history (Pharr et al., 2014).

According to varied sources (NAC and AARP, 2015) from 13% to 20% of African Americans are caregivers (most are women, but these figures usually are not broken down regarding age or gender, nor are they classified according to the situation of the caregiver, such as grandparents caring for grandchildren when the middle generation is absent). Also, numbers reflect those African Americans who have been included in research and define themselves as a *caregiver*, which is a technical term and which excludes an undetermined number of caregivers who either have not been part of a study or census, or do not call themselves caregivers. Of those African Americans who are recorded in caregiving polls, many (68%) are economically vulnerable and have lower life expectancy than White persons (Morano & King, 2010). Yet caregiving in communities of color is increasing and numbers are projected to triple by 2030 and quadruple by 2050 (Colby & Ortman, 2015; David, 2013; NAC & AARP, 2015) due to a projected African-American population growth within the next three decades, along with greater longevity in the African-American older population (Pharr et al., 2014). These projections present unique challenges for African Americans who are or may become caregivers, particularly African American elder males (David, 2013; Morano & King, 2010). One reason for this challenge is that African American elder male caregivers are considered most at-risk for psychological, social, and economic distress while assuming primary care for a loved one (Pharr et al., 2014). Yet they sometimes do not recognize (or admit) threats to personal well-being due to the amassed disadvantages experienced by older African American males born in the first half of the 20th century. Disadvantages include: having received inferior healthcare (particularly earlier in life), hazards inherent in available jobs when younger, and trauma incurred by discrimination, segregation, and racism during their lives (Mutua, 2006).

WHY WE WROTE THIS BOOK

This book addresses the gap in the gerontological literature on African-American older men who are the primary caregivers for loved ones. A reason for the lack of empirical knowledge on elder African-American male caregivers is that gerontological and health science studies have accomplished little research focused specifically on this group. Historically, African Americans mistrusted the process of research with good reason. Medical research had used vulnerable populations to perform painful medical tests (e.g., the Tuskegee syphilis studies and the Philadelphia Holmesburg Prison skin studies) or medical research done on African-American persons without their awareness that tests were performed and biological materials were taken (the case of Henrietta Lacks) or without being apprised of test results (Gelder, 2007; Jacobs, Rolle, Ferrans, Whitaker, & Warnecke, 2006). In other words, much research was unethical in nature.

When conducting social science research with African-American persons (or other marginalized groups), a potential to do harm exists by not sharing results with participants, by not showing how research findings aid the African-American community, or by attributing the findings of a small sample to a whole group (Black, Groce, & Harmon, 2011). Similarly, African Americans perceive research that asks solely for quantifiable answers as open to manipulation in analysis, and as "giving nothing back" to the African-American community, and causes reluctance to participate (Black et al., 2011). One of our caregiving respondents told us he was asked to participate in a telephone survey concerning political candidates' stand on healthcare issues. When asked to give a preset answer (yes, no, a lot, a little, not at all) to the questions asked, he declined to take the survey and informed the surveyor, "If you want my answers, you have to ask me the right questions." When *we* asked him to tell us the "right questions," he replied, "Questions that let me give my opinion; my answers have to take my history into account." We suggest that this crucial insight reveals the weight of history on present decisions, whether about caregiving or to participate in a research study, or to make a decision about "how to be" in a macro world in which African Americans continue to feel "outside" the domain of the dominant culture.

In light of "taking men's history into account" in interpreting responses to our questions, we offer a brief chronicle of men's communal pasts. We offer snapshots of critical episodes in African-American history and acknowledge their impact on the men who participated in our research. We disclose a glimpse of the large-scale context of African-American history in order to place men's caregiving behaviors on a historical continuum.

In acknowledging men's communal past, we note that their personal biographies and cultural backgrounds generate a worldview, and engender patterns of interpreting how global events in economics, politics, culture, and society affect the individual and community (David, 2013). Thus, an individual's past and present context are key to how he views and interprets present experiences.

HISTORY OF AFRICAN AMERICANS IN PHILADELPHIA

Momentous events, such as Slavery, Emancipation, Reconstruction, and the Great Migration of millions of Blacks fleeing the rural South to northern cities constituted the lives of African Americans for over three centuries. Crucial in the lives of African Americans since the Middle Passage were both their ancestors and "the five generations that follow us," as one respondent reported (Black et al., 2011). Men's history, as much as it included suffering and death inflicted *by* others, also bequeathed a legacy of giving care *to* others in order to aid the survival of African Americans as a people (Hines & Boyd-Franklin, 1996).

As we will see in later chapters, men who witnessed (as a child or young adult) family members giving care to an older adult, or themselves participated in caring for an aged or infirm relative or neighbor, became the primary caregiver for a loved one when needed. In fact, most men interviewed witnessed or took part in caregiving throughout their lives.

After emancipation from slavery in 1863 and during the years of reconstruction, southern Blacks, although labeled "free," remained economically and politically disenfranchised by the obstreperousness of southern lawmakers in disallowing Blacks economic and political autonomy. That is, constitutional amendments gave freedom to slaves (13th), made them citizens (14th), and gave Black males the right to vote (15th). Yet Jim Crow laws flourished, the Supreme Court struck down passage of the Civil Rights Act of 1875 (American Civil Rights Union, 2014), and the rise of the Ku Klux Klan subjected Blacks to ongoing violence and oppresion (Dees, 1991). One way for Blacks to extricate themselves from continued repression in the South was to head to the urban North in search of jobs and freedom. Philadelphia was one of the original major cities to which migrants flocked (Lane, 1991).

In the late 19th century at least two men collected information about the burgeoning population of Blacks in Philadelphia. In 1896, the University of Pennsylvania commissioned W. E. B. Du Bois to conduct a sociological study of African Americans in Philadelphia, including those who were born here and considered "elite," and those who migrated from the South (Lane, 1991). In 1899 the University of Pennsylvania published a compendium of Du Bois's "house-to-house case studies" entitled *The Philadelphia Negro*.

Another man, William Dorsey, an African-American historian born in 1837, was the son of an escaped southern slave who married a free White woman. The couple raised their family in Philadelphia. As a youngster, Dorsey witnessed the migration of Blacks who settled in Philadelphia. He amassed artifacts of Black life, such as news articles, pictures, stereotypes, and yarns about African Americans and eventually became custodian of the American Negro Historical Society. He noted that Philadelphia had become a nerve center for migrants. Information about available jobs and safe neighborhoods for Blacks was sent from Philadelphia to Washington and on to southern states where Blacks waited for word from family or friends to begin the trek north.

Dorsey's collection centered on Black life in the 19th and early 20th century. Through his artifacts, he illustrated the hardship Blacks endured by attempting to thrive in an adverse environment. In his journal, he named slavery as "the starting point" of the suffering he witnessed. "[Slavery] is the secular equivalent of original sin [and] the ultimate source of much of the tragedy of our history" (Lane, 1991, p. 3).

One caregiving man we interviewed gave an example of the distribution of practical information that continued to filter from Philadelphia to southern Blacks who were anxious to migrate in the mid-20th century. He recounted how migrants were warned about where to settle in Philadelphia.

> In the 1950s and '60s, when families came from down south, we told them, "Don't go above Arch and Race. Definitely don't go too far north; don't go to Northeast Philadelphia; that would be plain crazy." If you went to places where there were no Blacks, you were subject to scrutiny—or worse. You went into established Black neighborhoods, like South Philadelphia, that was the 7th Ward, or West Philly, where Blacks were confined to certain areas.

The 7th Ward in Philadelphia was remembered in a public art mural titled *Mapping Courage* by Carl Willis Humphrey in 2008. The mural was painted on the side of the 6th and South Streets fire station, memorializing the history of Engine 11, the 7th Ward, and W. E. B. Du Bois's research on African-American daily life in Philadelphia.

THE BLACK CHURCH

Another respondent described the Black Church as establishing the stability of Black neighborhoods; their pastors attempted to meet congregants' emotional, physical, and spiritual needs. He recounted the historical connection between the Black Church and the fight for freedom waged in the 18th century by slaves in Philadelphia.

> The center of the neighborhood was the Black Church. The church I grew up in was founded in 1792 by Absolom Jones. He and Richard Allen were slaves in 1760 and members of St. George's Methodist Church. The slaves could sit anywhere in the church like anybody else. Eventually St. George's wanted to build a bigger church and everybody helped—slaves and Whites. But after that the slaves were asked to sit somewhere else. When an usher asked Richard Allen and Absalom Jones to go to the balcony, they walked out. Richard Allen went on

> to found the Bethel African Methodist Episcopal Church (AME), and Absolom Jones founded St. Thomas Episcopal, where I'm still a member.

In researching this incident, several sources suggested that Richard Allen and Absalom Jones were "forcibly removed" from their seats in the church they helped build. The sad symbolism of this story centers on the diaspora—an ethnic group, removed from its homeland, forms a group identity based on their shared history of injustice and suffering (Cone, 1979). The Black Church crystallized this group identity in African Americans because of its distinctiveness as "African- and God-inspired as it stood in judgment upon the inhumanity of racism" (Wilmore, 1989, p. 244). The Black Church also showed broad parameters for redemption and salvation—health in body, mind, and spirit; and deliverance from evil in the secular (this world) and sacred (heaven) realms. Gaylord Wilmore (1989) noted that the pastors of Black Churches throughout history held a Bible in one hand and a newspaper in the other, cementing issues of political and social justice to religious belief and practice.

As we will see later in the book, men continued to look to their church for comfort and support throughout their lives, including periods of caregiving.

THE 20TH CENTURY

Our respondents were children, adolescents, and became adults in the first half of the 20th century. They lived during a period when legally sanctioned discrimination affected opportunities for education, housing, well-paying jobs, and voting rights. Integral to African-American men's hopes about achieving equality with Whites was laboring in the war effort, either by enlisting in the service or taking jobs that were open to Blacks in places like Philadelphia's army warehouse or the Navy yard (Black & Thompson, 2012).

The Selective Training and Service Act of 1940 prohibited discrimination by race in recruitment. Yet African-American World War II soldiers did not train, camp, or serve with White soldiers. For Black men who were wounded and needed blood transfusions, they received carefully separated blood that was labeled either "White" or "Black." When the war ended, segregated planes and trains took African-American soldiers home (Black & Thompson, 2012; Stouffer, 1949). African-American veterans returning from World War II were met with prewar discriminatory practices firmly entrenched. Angry and frustrated, they publicized the racist treatment they received during and after the war, which alerted the public and made issues of racism salient (Mutua, 2006).

A number of World War II veterans (Black and White) opted to remain in service at the end of World War II, and they later served in the Korean War (1950–1953) (Bowers et al., 1996). The executive order signed by President Truman in 1948 ordered all branches of the military desegregated. This order mandated equal treatment and access to opportunity for all servicemen, and made racist comments unlawful. The American History Archives (2015) noted that senior personnel often ignored these directives.

Some historians reported that fear of American tragedies on Korean battlefields actually brought integration into segregated military units. "The US military that went to Korea in 1950 was . . . looking squarely at defeat [due to sorely needed manpower]. With casualties mounting, segregation simply broke down" (AHA, 2015).

Fifty years later, in 2001, Colonel David J. Clark, director of the Korean War Commemoration Committee, called the situation of African-American soldiers in Korea: "both a tragedy and triumph. [It was] astonishing that they fought for others' rights while lacking [them] at home. It is a tragedy it occurred at all; a triumph that a fundamental injustice . . . began to turn the wheels of change in America" (Williams, 2001, p. 2).

African-American men served in Vietnam for reasons similar to those of World War II soldiers who had served their country 20 years earlier—they viewed military service as a forerunner to equality; it promised a better life in the postwar world (Beidler, 2000; Westheider, 1997). Despite integration of forces, research revealed a disparate experience for African-American servicemen due to (1) a disproportionate ratio of poor African-American men drafted into war to their percentage in the population (Westheider, 2003) and (2) continued racism experienced by African-American soldiers in Vietnam (Appy, 1997; see also the case of Mr. Gilmore in Chapter Four).

Although World War I, World War II, the Korean War, and the Vietnam War pioneered major social changes in American culture, the struggle for African Americans to be treated as equal members of society persisted. For example, military history of this era usually was recorded by White officers or military historians and therefore lacked an African-American perspective. Although African-American men had written articles and books about their service in the armed forces, the written materials were often printed privately and quickly went out of circulation (Black & Thompson, 2012).

We asked several of our respondents what they thought might be gained for African-American men in general by enlisting in the service. One veteran of the Korean War replied, "We placed our hopes in the United States. If we proved ourselves in the military, we would be part of the rehabilitation of the United States." Another man, a Buffalo Soldier veteran of World War II said, "After all, this was our country, too." As will be seen in a later chapter, several men in our study stated that the war in which they fought engendered suffering through racism and motivated them to return home as activists (Baldor, 2008; Black, 2015). (See the cases of Mr. Gilmore and Mr. Davis, Chapter Four.)

Despite hopes that enlistment would change African Americans' economic and social position in the United States, the 1950s witnessed the illogic and unconstitutionality of public schools as "separate but equal" in *Brown v. The Board of Education* in 1954, the courage and persistence of Blacks in the Montgomery Bus Boycott of 1955–1956, and the violence perpetrated on the Freedom Riders of 1960–1961 (PBS, 2015).

The 1960s witnessed ongoing rebellion among the poor, particularly African Americans and their advocates. This insurgence focused on lifelong unequal treatment in almost all aspects of daily life, including access to healthcare (Tumulty, 2014). The call for "jobs and freedom" led to the March on Washington in 1963 and its defining moment: the prescient speech given by Dr. Martin Luther King. He passionately noted that although Lincoln's Emancipation Proclamation had been signed 100 years previously, African Americans were obstructed from attaining their inalienable rights due to sanctioned racism by federal and state laws (Mutua, 2006). Despite various obstacles placed in the path of the March and against its leaders, President Kennedy invited Dr. King and March organizers into his office afterward, confirming his support of their goals (PBS, 2014). By doing so, he painted an imminent landscape of our country that, although indistinct, depicted a future that loomed brighter than the past. One of our respondents discussed his participation in the March wistfully:

> When I think back on being at the March in '63, if you stepped in front of someone, you said, "Excuse me." "Sure, that's all right." See, we realized what it meant, how important it was.

This man spoke to the reverential behavior of the marchers as actors in a momentous event. They realized that their participation—their words and actions—in the march, whether adulated or scorned, would be etched in America's history.

By 1964, there was a new president. President Kennedy had been assassinated the previous November, and a war that would divide the nation culturally and politically had begun in Southeast Asia. Yet the legacy of Kennedy's New Frontier became the national curriculum of the new president, Lyndon Johnson, which he named the Great Society. He signed the

Civil Rights Act in 1964, which made the unequal treatment of minority persons illegal. Using the metaphor of a battle to be won or lost, Johnson's War on Poverty promoted 40 programs intended to eliminate poverty by improving the conditions in which many people lived, particularly the aged and ill. For example, in 1964, despite Social Security, one out of three Americans over age 65 was living below the poverty line, largely due to medical bills (Tumulty, 2014). One of the Great Society's programs, the Older Americans Act of 1965, developed Medicare and Medicaid and guaranteed health care to all Americans over age 65 (Tumulty, 2014). Unfortunately, later administrations, including those of Nixon, Reagan, and Clinton, dismantled many of the programs that the War on Poverty had designed to assist those most in need.

Civil rights demonstrations continued across the country as the Vietnam War intensified. Both issues were symbols of the cultural and social fissures that ruptured America during the 1960s. African-American soldiers' recollections of Vietnam differed according to year of entry (Appy, 1993). At the beginning of the war, many African Americans supported its cause. By 1965 African-American soldiers, emulating Mohammed Ali questioned their involvement in fighting a dark-skinned enemy (Gallagher, 2014). In 1967, Martin Luther King denounced the Vietnam War, arguing that funds to finance it would be better used to aid America's poor (Beidler, 2000). After Dr. King's assassination in 1968, antiwar militancy grew stronger. In Vietnam and at home, a new consciousness of African-American identity engendered support for the Black Power movement. A growing consciousness of a powerful, shared Black identity emerged during this era. African Americans' frustration with the status quo and their desire for self-determination, buttressed by the support of Black clergymen, led to protests in American cities across the United States against systemic racism (Appy, 1993; Westtheider, 2003).

CAREGIVING

The psyche of African-American men as caregivers, their caregiving joys and burdens, and their relationship with friends and neighbors are rooted in their tragic and triumphant history. In the 20th century, an ill or infirm loved one was kept and cared for in the safety of an African-American home surrounded by family (whether persons were blood related or not). If economics or lifestyle did not permit caring for a loved one at home, there were few options in Philadelphia for poor African Americans to get adequate care (see Mr. Davis, Chapter Four), and there were fewer if any resources for treatment of the mentally ill.

For example, the Philadelphia Almshouse was Philadelphia's public hospital, nursing home, and home for the indigent. Opened in 1732, it operated under several names and was renamed Philadelphia General Hospital in the early 20th century. It was an institution where African Americans could access, as one of our respondents described, "the best treatment they could. It was less than the Whites had, but it was better than nothing." Philadelphia General became the hospital and home of ill, impaired, demented, or incarcerated persons who had no access to housing or care due to their ethnicity, low income, or lack of health insurance. Unfortunately, careless, unjust, or indifferent treatment toward the minority population put patients in peril. Insufficient staff and funding added to its grim reputation. The hospital was closed by Philadelphia Mayor Frank Rizzo in 1977; he believed that the passage of Medicare and Medicaid legislation (1965) would grant health insurance to the elderly and poor. Unfortunately, that did not occur; millions of disenfranchised persons without medical insurance were more vulnerable after passage of healthcare legislation (Rosenbaum, 2015).

The directors of Douglass Hospital and Mercy Hospital, separate entities until they merged in 1948, had hopes that the merged hospital, Mercy-Douglass, would become a "fully integrated institution . . . in which all groups, nationalities and races . . . work side by side" (Minton, 1951, p. 157). Mercy-Douglass Hospital, one of the oldest Black institutions in the city, closed in 1973, "a victim of mounting debts, lack of community support and changing times" (Beaver County Times, 1973).

The Home for the Aged and Infirm Colored Persons was founded in 1864 by wealthy Blacks and White Quakers who realized the hardship that slavery and discrimination posed for Blacks, and particularly for the aged. In 1953 the site became the Stephen Smith Home for the Aged, named for a wealthy Black merchant who contributed a large sum of money and property to the institution. Today, the Stephen A. Smith Home is a hospital and nursing home housing mainly African-American elders. It is located in West Philadelphia.

The history of our African-American elder caregiving men began in slavery, continued through emancipation, migration, military service, on to the civil rights movement and to the present day. For each respondent, an identity as an African-American man mapped particular meanings onto life experiences, such as religious affiliation, military service, getting married and becoming a father, and giving care to a loved one while growing old oneself. Men related throughout their interviews that all life experiences were filtered through eyes that held a panoramic sweep of a distant history of slavery and the recent chronicle of a lifetime troubled by discrimination, segregation, and racism.

There is an abiding irony in writing a book about African-American male caregivers. As Kramer and Thompson wrote in 2005, "There is an absence of research that focuses on ethnic variation in male caregiving" (p. 13). Until recently, if African-American men were included in research on male caregiving, they were either grouped with White male caregivers in order to measure, for example, *male* caregiver depression, role strain or satisfaction, or to be compared *to* White men for measuring ethnic outcomes on variables of caregiving. There was little understanding that for African Americans, there were no variables that could capture the integral nature of caregiving to their survival as a people (Pharr et al., 2014). In other words, there were few studies in which African-American elder male caregivers stood alone as participants in research that asked for their narratives about caregiving that also took their history into account.

We used an in-depth dialogical approach for our research (questions and answers become a dialogue between the interviewer and respondent). Although our questions were guided by an interview schedule, the interviewer followed the respondent's lead in the conversation. We enlisted the help of the community in undertaking this project. And although working within the community to study experiences within that community was not a new idea, the manner in which we conducted it was central to its success. All three authors and interviewers have been caregivers; two authors are African-American elder spousal caregivers. Because of this, there was an empathetic understanding between interviewer and respondent, and awareness that respondents' and interviewers' similar contexts, both biographical and historical, were key in our interpretation of their responses. The men whose reactions about caregiving were recorded in this book have a wealth of knowledge to offer those who have a professional or personal interest in the work and world of caregiving.

WHO WE ARE

The subject of "suffering" brought the authors together. The first author met the coauthors at a lecture that was held at a research hospital and university in Philadelphia. At the time, the first author co-conducted two studies on "The Experiences of Suffering in Old Age" (Rubinstein & Black, 1998). The first was a pilot study consisting of interviews with 40 elders about the subject of suffering. The second larger study consisted of 160 persons interviewed on the same topic. The first author interviewed her coauthors for the second study on suffering. The interviews began a journey that consisted of several writing projects; one became the authors' prior book: *From Zero to Eighty: Two African-American Men's Narratives of Racism, Suffering, Survival, and Transformation*, published in 2011. The interviews also resulted in an enduring friendship and partnership on in-depth research on various experiences in elder African-American men's lives.

Helen K. Black, PhD, has been a qualitative researcher for over 25 years. She has worked on federally funded projects researching experiences such as poverty among elders, forgiveness in old age, suffering in late life, caregiving daughters of demented mothers, African-American depression, life expectations in African-American older men, and the experiences of African-American veterans, among others. She is currently working on the subject of childlessness in elderly women and the experience of impaired adults attending adult day centers. She is the author of three other books: *Old Souls: Aged Women, Poverty, and the Experience of God*, with coauthor Robert Rubinstein, which was published in 2000, and *Soul Pain: The Meaning of Suffering in Late Life*, published in 2006. She recently completed an article on the generativity of the Oblate Sisters of Providence, who are religious sisters of color, and an article on African-American veterans of World War II, the Korean War, and the Vietnam War for *The Gerontologist*. She has authored five book chapters and over 40 articles in the fields of gerontology, African-American elders, qualitative research, issues of spirituality in age, and narrative studies. Until recently, Dr. Black was a caregiver in her home.

Dr. John T. Groce, EdD, MSW, has taught social work studies at Temple University, Lincoln University, Stockton College of New Jersey, and Widener University in Chester. He has decades of experience in the field of aging. At Catholic Social Services he was Administrator of the Migration and Refugee Services and Parish Social Ministry Department, where he directed social services for 40 city parishes. He was the supervisor for four senior centers run by the Archdiocese of Philadelphia. At the Philadelphia Corporation for Aging, he was a social worker in SARA, at the Information and Referral Department. He worked as a social worker with the Geriatric Mobile Mental Health Unit at the West Philadelphia Mental Health Consortium.

Dr. Groce is the cofounder of Mature Africans Learning from Each Other (M.A.L.E.), an organization that conducts workshops for African-American men and boys. Dr. Groce was married to Rosetta Anderson Groce for 60 years and was her primary caregiver until her passing. He has written several articles and lectured widely on issues relating to aging and African-American men and boys. His awards include Temple University General Alumni Association Certificate of Honor in 1990 and the Alumni Fellow Award in 2001.

Charles E. Harmon was educated in Philadelphia schools and graduated in 1949 from West Philadelphia High School. He spent 3 years at LaSalle College and attended two journalism schools. He worked in the US Post Office for 37 years. Through talent, hard work, and perseverance he realized his career goal of becoming a talk show host, newsman, and sports and street reporter for various Philadelphia radio stations, mainly WDAS, where he worked for 17 years. His radio shows were groundbreaking in the African-American community. He interviewed those who were "movers and shakers" in the government and entertainment industries, in the advancement of civil rights, along with the "common man or woman on the street" about issues important to African Americans. Charles Harmon is also a founding member of M.A.L.E. and has received numerous awards for community service. He has been married to Constance Harmon for 61 years.

John Groce and Charles Harmon have been friends for over 60 years. They are founders and members of area programs that encourage mature African-American men's (50+) community involvement. They have been long-time activists in their community, and they are often called upon to participate in workshops on various subjects affecting African Americans, to conduct seminars and clinics, to be guest lecturers in university classes, and to speak in various venues about the African-American elder experience, including the experience of the elder male caregiver. Their goal is to represent the African-American male as a role model and positive force in the life of his family, community, and culture. For this book, Groce and Harmon detailed the nature of research on male caregivers at practica, workshops, and church groups and requested participants for our study.

Thus, despite the history of African-American men's reluctance, mentioned previously, to be interviewed for research studies (Rexroth & Friedland, 2010), our respondents were willing to offer their caregiving experiences to the authors because the authors had lived through the same experiences. In return, we acknowledged each man's narrative for the treasure that it is.

A SHARED LABOR

The first author, in agreement with coauthors, planned the outline of the book and wrote the manuscript. The coauthors interviewed most of the men; the first author interviewed three respondents. Critical to the writing of the book was the coauthors' ability to describe the men they interviewed as well as their homes, neighborhoods, demeanor, and mood, and the insights and intuition they gleaned during visits. Also crucial to our work were the intangibles of interviewing that coauthors brought to this project: a deep understanding that comes from (1) being an African-American male with the shared history (with respondents) of growing up and coming of age in a segregated society; (2) residing in a large city with men who were born in the city or migrated from the South at an earlier age; and (3) having comparable caregiving experiences as the men they interviewed. In several ways, the coauthors' understandings and interpretations about caregiving were anchors for this book. The book could not have been written without close among the three of us.

The overarching question of our book is: What is the experience of being an elder African-American male caregiver? To construct a foundation for understanding the daily as well as long-term experience of caregiving, we asked the experts—a group of African-American male caregivers—to discuss the concrete and existential aspects of giving care to an ill or impaired loved one. Our book will begin to address what is missing from the literature about African-American male caregivers by revealing in case study form their experiences of life and of caregiving. (See Appendix A.)

The Hidden Among the Hidden

CHAPTER 1

Introduction

Informal male caregivers in general, or men who give unpaid care to a family member or friend in the home, have been considered "hidden" caregivers (Lane & King, 2012; Thompson, 2005). This "hiddenness" may be due to the constraints of masculinities, or behaviors that are considered appropriate for men, such as (1) hesitation to talk about the physical and emotional complexity of the caregiving situation, (2) reluctance to request help from healthcare agencies, and (3) a propensity to overlook one's own health problems due to time spent on caregiving tasks (HSC Foundation, 2010; Wong & Wallhagen, 2014).

Masculinities were epitomized in men's expectations of having control over self and circumstances in life situations, including caregiving. This depiction of control as typical behavior for men was said to influence their lack of expressivity about caregiving and reluctance to request help from either close others or formal groups (Black, 2010; Black, Schwartz, Caruso, & Hannum, 2008; Kramer & Thompson, 2005).

As mentioned, if male caregivers in general are considered "hidden" caregivers, elderly African-American male caregivers may be called "the hidden among the hidden." They are not only hidden as caregivers; they are hidden as men. There is negligible research on the older African-American male as an informal caregiver, and therefore the least amount of literature has been written about him (Thomas, 2012; Weinland, 2009). Outside of his own community, little is known about who he is, what his care work consists of, what gives him satisfaction in the role of caregiver and what he finds burdensome, and what meaning he finds in caregiving in the latter stages of life.

As more men in general assumed the hands-on tasks of informal caregiving, some men (1) proudly called themselves caregivers, (2) gained access to a healthcare system that supports them, and (3) were steered into research that learns from their experiences (Kramer & Thompson, 2008). National surveys provided estimates of the numbers of caregivers in the United States, the relation to the care recipient, the nature of tasks performed, hours spent in caregiving, and the duration of their care (NAC & AARP, 2015). Estimates presupposed that men defined themselves as caregivers when responding to surveys, which may not be the case. Some figures may have underestimated the care provided by men because they did not call themselves caregivers. Kramer and Thompson (2005) discussed the phenomenon of men's caregiving and the miscalculations made in surveys and census polls due to the subjective nature of defining care, caregiving tasks, and satisfaction gained or burdens levied when questions about caregiving required preset or one-word answers.

As the population ages, it is likely that among older men in general (more of whom are married due to high remarriage rates following divorce and widowhood), more husbands will take on the caregiving role for impaired wives. In recent surveys, men in the oldest old group (85+) were proportionately predominant in the caregiving role (Morano & King, 2010; USDHHS, 2011). Yet there is an absence of research that focuses on ethnic variation in this group (Pharr, Francis, Terry, & Clark, 2015). Thus, we know little about African-American caregiving men.

Our book presents in-depth portraits of caregivers who are considered the "hidden among the hidden." As we reveal their thoughts about caregiving, we offer readers entry into their worlds. Before we introduce the men who participated in our study on African-American male caregiving, we present a brief history of research and literature on informal caregiving in general.

BACKGROUND

Attention on Caregivers

In the 1960s healthcare professionals became aware of the growing numbers of persons, particularly those who were old, ill, and poor, who were cared for at home. Family members or friends who provided care for these persons were designated "informal caregivers." They assisted infirm loved ones with the activities of daily living and were not financially compensated for providing assistance (Vitaliano, Zhang, & Scanlan, 2003).

In the 1970s, and in the wake of the Older Americans Act, the attention of healthcare clinicians and researchers converged on probing the work and health of informal caregivers (Archbold, 1983; Mace & Rabine, 1981; Shanas & Streib, 1965; Troll, 1971). The changing nature of the family *who gives care* also came to light. A host of factors, such as fewer multigenerational households, adult children finding employment in distant cities and states, financial necessity for the informal caregiver to seek paid employment, along with the overwhelming nature of care tasks, brought caregivers' hidden work to light (Shanas & Streib, 1965; USDHSS, 2011). Until that time, informal caregiving was better known as "taking care of one's own" (Stewart, 2008). Many of us heard about or remember living in multigenerational family homes with grandparents and elder unmarried aunts and uncles. As elders became physically or cognitively infirm, they remained at home, cared for by family members (usually women) until they died.

Attention on family caregiving showed that caregivers' changing demographics spotlighted their value and emphasized the cost of losing their services. Replacing informal caregivers with formal services would place a financial strain on the healthcare system, as well as an enormous emotional toll on the care recipient and other family members (Kelly et al., 2008; Reinhard, Brooks-Danso, Kelly, & Mason, 2008).

The healthcare community's concern about informal caregivers increased and crucial questions arose: Who were they? Who became the primary caregiver of an impaired person and why? What type of care work did they perform? What kind of assistance would they seek from the healthcare system in order to continue caregiving? More questions followed: How burdensome was caregiving? How did it affect a caregiver's health? Did the caregiver find any satisfaction in caregiving? Answers to these questions were critical additions to extant formal data on informal caregiving (Reinhard et al., 2008).

Research on Caregiving

The major subjects of research on caregiving have been consistent. They are as follows: (1) the tasks informal caregivers perform, (2) managing difficult care-recipient behaviors, (3) caregiver burden, and (4) caregiver health. In fact, caregiver burden and its resultant effects on caregivers' health have framed a majority of caregiving research in the past decades (Dassel & Carr, 2016; Gaugler, Reese, & Mittelman, 2016; Pinquart & Sorensen, 2003).

Another significant topic in this literature are interventions designed to ameliorate caregiving burden in general (HSC Foundation, 2007) and in particular populations of caregivers such as vulnerable elderly spouses who are economically disenfranchised (Morano & King, 2010). Other topics include the common statistics of caregiving, such as the ever-increasing number of informal caregivers stratified and compared by age, ethnicity, gender, and tasks performed (Brummett & Dilworth-Anderson, 2012; Hasselkus & Murray, 2007; Kaufman & Tang, 2010; Mack, 2005; NCA & AARP, 2015).

The method of approach in researching these topics also has been consistent. For the most part, statistics reveal the demographics and background of informal caregivers, care recipients' level of impairment, the degree of stress experienced by caregivers, and their sense of satisfaction in caregiving (Kaufman & Tang, 2010; NAC & AARP, 2015). Much of this work has been theorized using a stress and coping model that emphasizes negative aspects of caregiving (such as emotional or physical distress) and factors (such as support networks or personal resilience) that mediate caregiving burden (Kelly, Reinhard, & Brooks-Danso, 2008; Morano & King, 2010). We note that numbers in the caregiving literature vary, depending on sources cited, such as census surveys and caregivers' associations, and the field of study under which the study is conducted, e.g. nursing, gerontological studies, or social work (Gaugler et al., 2016; Levine, 2008).

Some of the latest research on elder caregiving reported in top-tier gerontological journals showed that researchers used large secondary data sets to glean caregiving trends. From these sources researchers learned that: (1) dementia caregiving accelerates frailty in caregivers (Dassel & Carr, 2016); (2) caregiving is a productive activity for elders that "may reduce [their] bodily inflammation" (Kim & Ferraro, 2014)" and (3) spousal caregiving "is not uniformly associated with compromised well-being" (Freedman, Cornman, & Carr, 2016).

Despite these contradictory findings, studies agree on one caregiving fact: family caregivers remain indispensable to their smaller family world and to the larger healthcare system (Reinhard et al., 2008). Research showed that because informal caregivers provided close to 90% of all home care for the ill and impaired, they saved the state and federal governments millions of dollars in costs by assuming the role of primary support for vulnerable loved ones (Dassel & Carr, 2016; Scharlach, 2008). The increased longevity of Americans became key in the growing societal awareness of the work of caregiving. The number of impaired elders rose along with the growing number of older Americans in general (Reinhard et al., 2008). As baby-boomers reached 65, the number of caregivers who themselves were elders also increased. These facts raised the likelihood that a caregiver who was over 60 years of age was giving care to more than one family member, such as an elderly parent and a spouse, and endured his or her own health problems due to aging (Kelly et al., 2008; USDHHS, 2011). When married couples were caregiver and care recipient, both were considered vulnerable older adults (Scharlach, 2008).

In the last decade, professional support services that once assisted caregivers became more informational and managerial rather than clinical or actively supportive. Thus, at the same time that individual caregivers were offered less clinical assistance from professional caregiving agencies (Dassel & Carr, 2016; Kelly et al., 2008), technological assistance for caregivers has burgeoned. Various online classes, support groups, and interventions for caregivers are offered, which assumes that caregivers own computers and are literate in the language (Adler & Mehta, 2014; Daniel, Deering, & Murray, 2014; Gaugler et al., 2016; Morano & King, 2010).

WHO IS THE CAREGIVER?

The picture of the most common caregiver was a middle-aged woman who might be caring for two elders—an elder parent, parent-in-law, spouse, or other older relative. She often worked outside the home, had children of her own and also grandchildren for whom she cared, but continued to accomplish the affective and instrumental tasks of caregiving (AARP, 2009). Research showed that close to 70% of informal caregivers are women (Given, Sherwood, & Given, 2008; NAC & AARP, 2015; United States Department of Health and Human Services, 2011). The reality of this caregiving picture also was based on a cultural construction that care work was women's work (Calasanti & King, 2007). The word *caregiver* connoted the traditionally feminine characteristics of nurturance and sustenance. "Let's face it," one man interviewed for this book commented, "even at our best we can't hold a candle to the women."

Yet over 30% (some sources put the figure closer to 40%) of caregivers were male, often an elderly spouse who was caring for a wife with some form of dementia (NCA & AARP, 2015; USDHHS, 2011). Although women still provided the bulk of family care, the number of male caregivers providing hands-on care to loved ones, particularly spouses, grew. Although male caregivers seemed overshadowed by the feminization of caregiving and by the numbers of female caregivers, the picture of the caregiver evolved as more men assumed the role (Scharlach, 2008).

Caregiving—A Gendered Phenomenon

In the gerontological literature a standard picture of the male caregiver was a European-American man who was both silent and hidden. He was considered comfortable with the practical, instrumental, and nonaffective tasks of caregiving, such as handling whatever "equipment" caregiving entailed, such as installing bathtub pulls, lifting the wheelchair, or managing finances. The actual "body" work, or the touch of caregiving, was accomplished by women. When a man spoke about caregiving, either because he requested help from a formal agency or joined a support group, he was lauded. He even may have gained some recompense in the form of praise from outsiders or family members for having performed the all-encompassing and exhausting role of caregiver (Kramer, 2005).

Who was the male caregiver? As mentioned previously, he was often described as an elderly spouse taking care of a wife who suffered from a cognitive or physical impairment (NAC & AARP, 2015; Russell, 2007). One description of him was that he was reversing roles with his wife as he performed caregiving tlasks (Hanlon, 2012; Kramer & Thompson, 2005). Meal planning, cooking, and cleaning, once his wife's domain, was accomplished by an elderly husband with, at times, help from an adult child, a paid caretaker, or both. Yet monitoring the health and well-being of a demented or disabled spouse did not necessarily become easier with years of practice. In a previous study, one male caregiver succinctly spoke about caring for his wife, who suffered from mid-stage Alzheimer's disease, as he faced the future: "With Marie [wife], it don't, it won't get better. It just gets deeper" (Black et al., 2008).

The Caregiver's "Lived Experience"

In this book, we viewed the daily intricacies of African-American elder male caregivers' work and life with the care recipient as "lived experiences." The term "lived experience" (*erleben*) is borrowed from German philosophy (Husserl, 1964). According to its origin, the term connotes what an individual lives through and experiences personally and immediately. A lived experience also includes the persisting content of that experience. That is, the residue of the experience that remains after the event has passed (Desjarlais & Throop, 1997; Gadamer, 1975).

Reactions to a lived experience are gender based and contextual. Individuals learn to experience or endure a situation as a male or female at a particular place in time (Lotterhos, 2015; Martin, 1987; Russell, 2007).

Masculinity and femininity are social constructs that advocate distinct behaviors for men and women. The cultural impetus for men and women to act in accordance with gender roles is internalized throughout life (Thompson, 2005). When aged male caregivers were growing and developing, society upheld a set of attitudinal and behavioral roles and rules for men and women (and different roles and rules for African-American men and women) (Calasanti & King, 2007). What became customary in a society (such as women are natural caregivers) became a "taken for granted" or universal cultural idea. Thus, individuals' actions related to caregiving were informed by gender-appropriate responses that family and society tacitly and overtly assigned (Mirowsky & Ross, 1995).

Feminine characteristics of nurturance and sustenance were interwoven with women's major roles as wife, mother, and caregiver (Martin, 1987). As defenders and protectors of family and country, men believed that they should be strong, unemotional, and, for the most part, silent about negative experiences, such as war, poor health, and caregiving (Hanlon, 2012). These masculine behaviors are rooted in the American concept of the person as a hero (Bellah, Madsen, Sullivan, Swidler, & Tipton, 1985; Pierre, Mahalik, & Woodland, 2001), whose central story is that of the quest, in which the hero overcomes myriad dangers. This model of self-directed action embodied by the hero is linked to moral correctness and control over life circumstances. Autonomy, privacy, and responsibility are key characteristics (Bellah et al., 1985; Black & Thompson, 2012; Mutua, 2006; Ribeiro, Paul, & Noguiera, 2007). The hero is outwardly directed; his battles are waged in the world of combat, competition, and resistance. Although women have kept the "feminine" characteristics mentioned earlier, they also have taken on the qualities of the "hero" (Martin, 1987) in light of women's evolving views about themselves and the multiplicity of their roles. In Chapter Seven, we explore caregiving as a pilgrimage that the caregiver, care recipient, family, and community travel together, rather than the solo journey of the hero.

The "hero," even as he grows old, does not relinquish masculinities. The importance of physical strength, pushing oneself to the limit, and remaining stalwart while in pain might engender a bracketed (an individual separates himself from the feelings of a negative experience) reaction to the effort of caregiving. Or men might view the tasks of caregiving as external problems to fix or solve, often privately (Kramer, 2005; Thompson, 2005).

In other facets of men's lives, such as health and safety, masculinities have been viewed as potential detriments to men's well-being. That is, men may work too hard or engage in risky behaviors in order to achieve a certain material goal, such as wealth, a reputation as being hard-nosed, or simply keeping one's job because succumbing to pain might be construed by others as weakness (Black, 2001; Courtenay, 2000; Mutua, 2006; Pierre, Mahalik, & Woodland, 2001).

Having a casual attitude toward personal health might apply to the male caregiver. For example, although he realizes that living through the "36-hour day" (Mace & Rabine, 1981) of caregiving is a monumental task, he may refuse help or not request it. Thus, the overwhelming nature of caregiving reveals the underside to the masculine ideal, which might be hesitancy to admit feeling overwhelmed (Ribeiro, Paul, & Nogueira, 2007). He might perceive seeking relief from daily chores as "unmanly." A sense of loss of control over one's work, in this case, caregiving, collides with the self-reliance men consider a fixed part of their identity (Russell, 2007).

According to ethnographic interviews conducted with male and female caregivers of various ages, a hallmark of informal caregiving was to feel unprepared for the intense labor of caregiving and the negative effect of the care recipient's impairment on the caregiver's mood and personality (Black et al., 2008). Yet, for male caregivers, requesting help may resonate with vulnerability. Even sharing a sense of burden with someone who has gone through similar crises may be thought as "whining or looking for sympathy" (Black, 2010).

One elderly man whose wife had a variety of illnesses, including dementia, reported that she was "acting paranoid." She thought neighbors were entering their home through the roof and stealing her clothes. This behavior so upset him that he mentioned it to a neighbor who also was a caregiver to a wife with dementia.

> When my wife got sick, I said something to the guy across the street. I told him I felt pretty bad. His wife was sick, too. He didn't say much, so I didn't say anymore. I didn't want to burden him.

Although this man attempted to reach out to someone who might understand his circumstances, the other man's initial reticence caused him to retreat. There is poignancy in the image of two long-time neighbors, having shared decades' worth of experiences as homeowners, fathers, and aged caregivers, unable to converse about the subject that most affected their later years (Black, 2006).

Are men usually reticent on the subject of caregiving? Perhaps it depends on a caregiver's notion of privacy, his perception of appropriate gender roles, suitable reactions to hardship or loss, the meaning of illness, impairment, and personhood, and whether anyone asks questions about his caregiving experiences (Black, 2006; Kitwood, 1997; Thompson, 2005).

Viewing gender identity as a social construction reveals that it can be deconstructed and rebuilt (Martin, 1987). Like a concrete cultural artifact, gender identity can be reinterpreted in light of caregiving. When viewed as a changeable construct, gender identity becomes fluid and shaped by the context and needs of the caregiver and care recipient rather than a strict external posture (Brandtstadter & Greve, 1994). Male caregiving challenges the fixedness of a normative system of gender behaviors, and precipitates a clash with long-held perceptions of masculinities (Courtenay, 2000; Thompson, 2005). Through the work of caregiving, an elderly man might ponder the question: What must I do, think, and become in the latter stages of life in order to take on or continue the work of caregiving? (Given, Sherwood, & Given, 2008). In the next chapter we will meet a caregiver who asked this question of himself.

African-American Male Caregivers

Although more research on elderly African-American male caregivers has been called for, there are few works that provide this internal view from the perspective of African-American caregivers (Moore, 2010; Thomas, 2012; Weinland, 2009). It is for this reason that we sought the real experts of African-American elder male caregiving—the men themselves.

It is important to place our work and the African-American men we interviewed in context. Here, the broad context is the macro world of a society constructed and structured by top-down implicit norms and rules about aging, ethnicity, ability, manhood, and life roles. The context also includes men's micro world, which is equally constructed and structured by family and community beliefs and traditions. Another significant aspect of African-American caregivers' context is history, both distant and recent.

W. E. B. DuBois wrote in *The Souls of Black Folks* (1903b) that African-American identity suffers through the rupture of a "double consciousness," or by perceiving two identities within the self. One identity is created through the reflections of trusted others and shows the self as authentic. The other identity is created through the ethos of the dominant culture and has shown the African-American male as "less than" in the wider society. If this worldview is internalized, the result is a fissured sense of self. Yet there is little phenomenological material on the experience of double consciousness of African-American men juxtaposed with both caregiving and American idealized masculinities (Mutua, 2006). We acknowledge that perhaps an insidious aspect of the "double consciousness" theory is that it presupposes a standard of self-integration that hypothetically exists in European-American men.

We suggest that African-American men's masculinities continue to be shaped by societal contradictions. That is, they were framed both by the realities of African-American life and the myth of the "hero." The dominance of the hero clashed with society's built-in deficits against African-American males. Most African-American men, particularly those born in the first half of the 20th century, felt constrained by this double-bind situation, in which conflicting instructions about African-American manhood can render many problems insoluble. As mentioned, the lived experience of being an African-American caregiver who does not trust the healthcare community and is hesitant to request help may be especially at risk for both mental and physical stresses due to caregiving. Despite this, there is little phenomenological material on the double consciousness of African-American caregivers juxtaposed with American idealized masculinities (Pierre et al., 2001).

We acknowledge that African-American culture and society is heterogeneous and discloses great diversity. Yet a group's cultural framework incorporates the sum of its experiences, including those of the long past, such as slavery, sharecropping, and Jim Crow, into its current norms and values (Pharr, Francis, Terry, & Clark, 2014).

One of our goals in discussing African-American men as caregivers is to challenge the "deficit" view of African-American culture, society, and family life (Hines & Boyd-Franklin, 1996), particularly the experiences of the African-American elder male (Groce, 2002). We attempt to bring a more balanced depiction of African-American strengths in the face of discrimination that marked daily life for our respondents while they were young, and although less overt, continued as they matured.

We show that African-American life, viewed in light of its positive legacies, must be refracted in terms of its "collective unity, extended family systems, spirituality, and pride in its heritage (Hines & Boyd-Franklin, 1996, p. 67). It also must be refracted through (1) the memory of the history of suffering which is deeply internalized within the psyche of African Americans (David, 2013); (2) the lack of dialogue *by all Americans* about the varied effects of distant and recent history *on all Americans*, and (3) the racism that continues into the twenty-first century. Continuing racism appears as everyday micro-aggression or deadly hostility, both of which disclose what lies beneath the gloss of political and social correctness (Solorzano, Ceja, & Yosso, 2000; Wing Sue, 2010).

As previously mentioned, despite the scope of research on caregiving, there is scant research on African-American male caregivers (Thomas,

2012). The development of African-American caregiving behavior largely resulted from African Americans' distant history of slavery and their forced journey to foreign lands, and the more recent history of racism in America (Mutua, 2006; Pierre et al., 2001). African-American ancestors giving care to one another shaped the configuration of African-American family life. Their marginalized circumstances in America guided the formation of prosocial, generative behaviors to kin and nonkin (Dilworth-Anderson, Goodwin, & Williams, 2004; Gilkes, 1997; Mattis et al., 2007). In fact, African Americans used fluid definitions of family to describe their caregiving relationships, such as informal adoption, shared childrearing, having fictive or play kin, and giving kin-like care to nonbiological others (Janevic & Connell, 2001; Mattis & Jaggers, 2001; Mattis et al., 2007). Necessity also forced generative attitudes and behaviors toward strangers. History revealed that food and shelter, along with physical and mental healthcare, became the community's shared responsibility and was assumed particularly by the Black Church (Mattis & Jaggers, 2001; Raboteau, 1978). Due in part to marginalization by the dominant society, African American women *and* men were socialized to provide care for the "other," whether or not the other was biologically related or even well known to the caregiver (Dilworth-Anderson et al., 2004).

Several of our respondents, when asked if they called themselves a caregiver, answered, "No." They described themselves instead as "just a loving husband" or "devoted son" and "doing what I'm supposed to do." In light of this, another picture of the caregiver emerges. Ten percent of African Americans in the United States are caregivers (USDHHS, 2011). As mentioned previously, this figure may be grossly underestimated due to the fact that many African-American men may not call themselves caregivers. Traditionally, informal care was the primary way that African-American aged and infirm adults received assistance for the tasks of daily living (Dilworth-Anderson et al., 2004; Hopp & Thomas, 2014).

Many caregivers (68%) both male and female are economically vulnerable. And, although African Americans continue to have lower life expectancy rates than do European Americans, Hispanics, and Asian Americans, the life expectancy of African Americans is increasing along with their population numbers (HSC Foundation, 2007). The number of African-American older adults who will need some manner of care is expected to triple by the year 2030. This estimate presents a specific challenge for African-American older adults and their families.

Changed patterns in African-American families, including the migration of adult children to another state for attending school or finding employment, will render the elder spouse the primary and sole caregiver for an ailing or demented husband or wife (Anderson & Turner, 2010; HSC Foundation, 2007; Moore, 2010; Thomas, 2012; Weinland, 2009).

As mentioned, the African-American elder male caregiver has been considered the most vulnerable of caregivers in recognizing his own psychological, social, and economic distress while being the primary caregiver for a loved one (Anderson & Turner, 2010; HSC Foundation, 2007). His concern about whether he is doing the "job" well adds to the stress of his labor. One man interviewed for this book said,

> It's not just that I'm reversing roles with Charlotte (wife), it's that I have to keep on building on it. She doesn't always tell me what I need to know [to cook meals or do laundry properly]. I have to figure it out myself.

Another caregiver reported that his wife

> . . . made the best fried chicken I ever tasted. When she got sick, I asked her how to make it, told her I'd make it for her. She said, "I don't know." I put it to jealousy. She didn't want me to know how to make it. But I never put it to dementia. We take what they say, even when they sick, that they in good mental health. So I found myself denying that her lack of cooperation was due to dementia.

This "building on" work of caregiving sometimes meant facing an impaired care recipient's inability to perform the tasks in which she excelled or to articulate her "how-to" of accomplishing the tasks to the caregiver. It also sometimes entailed confronting a demented care recipient's resentment about sharing her knowledge and skills. As the earlier participant noted about his wife, "She didn't want me encroaching on her territory; [she didn't want] to lose control of running her domain."

Another African-American man interviewed in a prior study (Black et al., 2008), who we called Mr. Adams, described his response as "strong-willed" when his wife was first diagnosed with Alzheimer's disease. "If I set my mind to do something, I'm determined to do it. Because no matter what happens I'll take care of her. And if it's possible to beat it . . . but I had no idea how drastic it was."

In fact, this man's response was typical of the African-American male caregivers we interviewed. Although determined to do the job alone, few foresaw the consuming and progressive nature of the loved one's illness (particularly Alzheimer's disease and related dementias), the tasks of caregiving, and the unforgiving effects of making a mistake while giving care. Mr. Adams continued:

> One morning we came down the steps and got to the last two. She held the railing and I'm in front of her. If she fell, I would catch her. She let go and slid

> down. I tried to catch her, but I must have hit her in the rib. She cried out. I was frightened and I was very, very, very upset and it was like I was going to come apart. That was a turning point. Because when she fell, she hit her head, not her rib. How did it happen? I concluded I did it.

Mr. Adams was overcome with fear and guilt. After the fall, the couple's bed was brought into the dining room; his wife no longer used the stairs. Mr. Adams's account also suggested that common, everyday actions, such as "coming down to breakfast," possessed both enormous power as well as peril in the couple's shrinking world (Black et al., 2008).

The paradox of caregiving was effectively portrayed by Mr. Adams. He spoke of his most salient characteristic as an African-American man—determination—fostered by his family of origin and honed by discrimination he endured at work. He reported that he pushed his career forward "despite setback." Yet his resolve could not help him "beat her [wife's] sickness."

No statistical scales could adequately measure the depth of emotion with which Mr. Adams recounted his wife's fall or his ongoing devotion to her. Throughout the interview, he reiterated that even when she no longer speaks to him "or even opens her eyes," he will "be happy that she's here." His desire to repay *her* love throughout their lives remained a major impetus for caregiving.

SUFFERING

In the study on suffering mentioned earlier, "Experiences of Suffering in Later Life" (Black & Rubinstein, 2004), two older African-American men (N = 80) were caregivers for impaired wives. Each man reported that caregiving included experiences of personal suffering. The reasons included (1) the physical pain and potential injury that resulted from having to lift or turn someone who is either resistant or dead weight; (2) the uncertainty of what the next phase of the disease might bring; (3) the anticipatory grief of an expected death (Black, 2006; Chapman & Pepier, 1998; Holley & Mast, 2009), and (4) the mourning that occurs when an elderly loved one becomes ill with dementia (Black, 2010).

In the present study, one respondent described his wife's cognitive impairment as

> . . . suffering. I don't know whether she realizes it (that she is cognitively impaired). Sometimes I believe she does, but then I can't say. But if she does, or realizes it some of the time, that must be suffering.

He described his own suffering as "the loss of [his wife] as she used to be." This suffering also caused a specific type of mourning, which is neither anticipatory grief nor grief due to death. We discuss this kind of mourning in a later chapter.

A sense of control over self and life circumstances is also considered a "life value," the loss of which was named suffering by many study participants in the study on suffering (Black, 2006, 2011; Black & Rubinstein, 2004). Related closely to masculinities, control refers to having a sense of freedom in initiating and carrying out personal choices (Morling & Evered, 2006; Skinner, 1996). Having some "say" over the circumstances of one's life, no matter how diminished by illness, caregiving, or the long-term effects of discrimination, has been identified as a coping strategy in relation to caregiving *and* to suffering (Black et al., 2008). When the caregiver is an elderly African-American man, exercising autonomy over the range of care tasks performed revealed competency as both a man and a caregiver (Ribeiro, Paul, & Nogueira, 2007).

Research on the subject of suffering found that experiences of suffering often hurled a predictable world into chaos. The small purposes of daily living (such as family, work, friendships, and interests) that merged into an individual's larger sense of purpose were disrupted during suffering (Becker, 1997; Charmaz, 1999). Suffering was described as a rupture of the self, occurring from loss of roles and confusion about identity (Becker, 1997; Charmaz, 1999), assaults to the self's wholeness, and fear of death (Cassell, 1982). Would our African-American male caregivers describe experiences of caregiving as suffering?

NARRATIVE

For the men interviewed, narratives of caregiving had moral and social significance (Given et al., 2008). They were narrated by men who, while growing and developing, were marginalized in the larger world, yet socialized to care for needful members of the community (Mattis & Jaggers, 2001). Their narratives represented the "right way" to be. An important aspect of respondents' narratives highlights the reciprocity of giving care, especially in the case of caregiving husbands (Courtenay, 2000). Our respondents often gave a variation of one man's thoughts about the reciprocal nature of caregiving: "She has taken care of me throughout our lives; it's right that I take care of her now." Most narratives included pieces of the care recipient's biography as well as accounts of present or recent caregiving, which showed the continuity of their lives through time. Even after the loved one's death, the caregiver continued to interpret the caregiving experience as meaningful; it gave enduring worth to the care recipient's personhood through his memory of her (Black, 2006).

Narratives of caregiving often show the harsh realities of our world, such as illnesses that have no cure, the mystery of personhood in dementia, and the helplessness of those who watch and give care. Offering a narrative about caregiving in the latter stages of life may serve as a latter chapter in the caregiver's end-of-life story. It is often the caregiver's final, physical act of love, as well as his last "career" (Black et al., 2008). Some of the men's narratives assumed aspects of a life review, with the present labor of caregiving woven retrospectively into a personal history. For example, knowing that caregiving was a central aspect of his story, the spousal narrator often added to the narrative the sacrifices his wife made through the years, equalizing their relationship with present or recent caregiving. An essential feature of most caregiving narratives included the complex nature of mature, reciprocal love with the humbling and humanizing aspects of old age and illness. In the African-American community, caregiving itself was the language that two individuals, the caregiver and care recipient, spoke to each other, as the community watched, listened, and learned.

METHODOLOGICAL FRAMEWORK

We used narrative inquiry, a form of qualitative research, as the method of eliciting responses from our participants. The qualitative questionnaire, which was semistructured and included open-ended questions as well as basic demographics, was the main tool of our study (see Appendix A). The questionnaire was crafted by the authors to include queries that would ultimately address the main topic of our study: the experience of being an elder African-American male caregiver. From answers to this questionnaire, we produced an ethnographic narrative of each of our participants, or a portrait of 13 elder African-American men as caregivers, in as complete a picture of them and the care recipient as possible.

Ethnography means "writing a portrait of a people." It is a written depiction of a group that comprises a particular ethos, in their own setting. Here, the ethos or culture that the group shares is that they are African-American elderly male caregivers. The setting is each man's home, neighborhood, and urban community. Our qualitative methodology considers our male caregivers as the experts of the reality of their lives, and best able to explain the history of their caregiving. Their "reality" forms the guidelines for authors' interpretations of men's responses.

Through this method of narrative inquiry, we discovered how a caregiver was oriented to caregiving by seeking the biography of his caregiving *and* the meaning of his caregiving role (Van Manan, 1990). We were able, with caregivers' assistance, to decipher the complex emotions involved in caregiving and to interpret the relationship with the care recipient. We were especially attuned to respondents' expert insight regarding the influence of culture and ethnicity on the experience of caregiving.

Recent literature supports the position that the cultural values that an individual brought to caregiving were complex and could not be interpreted by a single construct, model, or paradigm (Scharlach, 2008). Our methodology provided opportunities for men to express a nuanced articulation of the values they brought to caregiving without attempting to place their experiences under preset categories. Instead, *their responses* produced the categories or themes of this book. Narrative inquiry revealed the cognitive and emotive processes behind caregivers' interpretations for why they gave care. Our method also used prompts and probes in interviewing so we might reach multileveled understandings of caregivers' use of ambiguity, nuance, metaphor, and symbolism. Men's responses to prompts, probes, and tailor-made follow-up questions expanded men's range of expression about caregiving.

The use of qualitative methods to obtain data in this study was crucial due to African-American elders' well-documented comfort with dialogical research (Rexroth & Friedland, 2010) in which they can narrate an account of their past, their current experience, and their expectations and goals. Our approach acknowledged not only the strong oral tradition in African-American culture (Raboteau, 1978) but also African-American's men's history of *not* being asked for their opinions or having their viewpoint taken seriously, and the significance of each man's voice telling *his own* story.

Design

This book used data collected from a research study on African-American male caregivers that explored the experience and meaning of being an elderly male caregiver. We qualitatively interviewed 13 caregivers. The private, two-session interview lasted approximately 2 hours in each session, for a total of 4 hours with each respondent.

Inclusion Criteria

Included in this study were African-American male caregivers, aged 60 and above. All respondents were (1) English speaking, (2) cognitively intact, and (3) able and willing to engage in two, 2-hour interview sessions about caregiving.

Respondents

We recruited our sample of African-American caregiving men from the community outreach of the authors. We note that qualitative sampling is purposive rather than random (Strauss & Corbin, 1990). Thus, in order to provide readers with in-depth portraits of caregivers, we chose to interview 13 men living in the Philadelphia community who were known as caregivers to Groce and Harmon. This number is both an adequate sample size in qualitative terms and manageable in terms of our ability to represent each man in our book as expansively as possible (Luborsky & Rubinstein, 1995). We purposefully recruited African-American elder male caregivers who were able and willing to talk about their caregiving experiences in the past and present. In the present sample, all men were over 60 years of age. The youngest man was aged 62 and the oldest, 87, with the average age being 75 years. All men hailed from the working classes; all had attained at least a high school education; three men had advanced degrees. Although all men responded positively when asked if they were either religious or spiritual, not all men reported that they belonged to a particular religious denomination. Of those who did, four men said that they were Baptist, two were Catholic, one was Presbyterian, and two were Muslim. Most of the men were long-married, and all had given care to a loved one at home for at least 5 years and as long as 30 years. Some of the men cared for more than one person at the same time; a few of the men cared for more than one person at different times. Their loved ones endured a variety of illnesses and debilities that necessitated hands-on care.

Our book examines several aspects of the caregiving experience, including the perception each man holds of himself, the unique generativity of African-American men who are caregivers, the suffering endured during caregiving, the mourning that occurred before and after the care recipient's death, the significance of support during caregiving, the import of men's friendship with other men, men's religiousness and spirituality, and the emotions, conflicts, and choices that emerge in the daily care routine.

Table 1.1 shows the name and age of each caregiver, years spent caregiving, the person for whom he cared, and a representative quote about caregiving.

Data Collection

We base our narrative portrait of African-American caregiving men on several items of collected data: (1) two digitally recorded semistructured qualitative interviews, which were processed through transcription; (2) field notes created by each interviewer, which included a description of the caregiver, his home and neighborhood environment, the caregiver's demeanor in relation to the entire interview, and in some cases, in relation to questions he did not answer or what he did not say during an interview; and (3) field notes of team meetings, which were held as close to once weekly as possible with all team members (authors and transcriptionist) attending. Team meetings had several purposes. Each caregiver was discussed as a case study (Flyvbjerg, 2006), with the person who conducted the interview presenting interpretations of the case, and other team members asking questions and at times offering alternative interpretations. In meetings, we also discussed the suitability of questions; for example, did any question elicit little response or seem confusing to the respondent and, if so, how should the question be altered for future interviews. In team meetings, all team members had the opportunity to share insights and intuitions about respondents and interviews, respondents' similarities and differences, and themes and patterns that emerged in their answers.

The Institutional Review Board from the first author's university approved the ethical conduct of the project. Interviewers audio-recorded a statement of information about the project (the study was for research purposes, each participant's right to confidentiality and anonymity, as well as to not answer any question deemed unacceptable for any reason, or to end the interview at any time and for any reason) and requested consent from each participant at the start of the first interview. Also recorded were participants' responses of consent. Data collected for this project, including interview questionnaires, transcripts, and field and meeting notes, were kept in a locked file in the first author's locked office. All identifiers on collected data were removed; all respondent materials were given a project number.

Table 1.1: NAME AND AGE OF EACH CAREGIVER, YEARS SPENT CAREGIVING, THE PERSON FOR WHOM HE CARED, AND A REPRESENTATIVE QUOTE ABOUT CAREGIVING.

Caregiver	Age	Care Recipient	Time Giving Care	Representative Quote
Bill Abbott	82	Wife Charlotte	25 years	I mourn the old Charlotte. I mourn her every time I look at her and she's out of it.
Horace Brunson	70	Wife Mattie Wife Barbara	5 years 4 years	When I tell somebody something, I want to live to that fully. The one thing I do despise is liars.
Louis Colbert	62	Mother	4 years	She knew you were a male relative, but not who. Then you'd hold her and she'd put her head on your shoulder and she'd relax 'cause she knew she was safe. That was important—knowing she felt safe and not in pain.
Elliot Davis	87	Wife Gemma	10 years	It got to the point—and I think that's where frustration set in with me. A simple thing became difficult—like taking the wheelchair out of the car.
Alexander El	68	Mother Mother-in-law	3 years 4 years	My mom was the shoe and I was the laces.
Eddie Gilmore	64	Wife Donna	6 years	They say, "You stood up as an Afro-American and you are an inspiration." I said, "It's there—black men *are* taking care of their spouses."
Claude Gross	79	Mother	5 years	Me and her was really tight, and so for 5 years she was in the Alzheimer's thing. But it took a while for me to pick that up, what was happening.
James Kelch	76	Wife Beverly	4 years	You know it'll be 17 years this December that she's been gone. It doesn't seem that long. I don't know how I've lasted this long without her. I never thought I would outlive her.
Ellis Moore	76	Wife	4 years	I said, "Don't send anybody (aides) anymore." So I kind of learned to cook and she could kind of tell me what to do with the stuff, you know. I ain't never been no cook.

(continued)

Table 1.1: Continued.

Caregiver	Age	Care Recipient	Time Giving Care	Representative Quote
Fred Parker	76	Wife Mother	2 years	I felt more as a needed husband than a caregiver. She needed me to do this. After she passed my mother got sick. I brought her here and it was almost the same pattern.
Harry Stokes	83	Mother	4 years	I didn't see myself as a caregiver. I saw myself as the son that's supposed to do what he's supposed to do for his mother.
Charles Wayns		Wife Mother-in-law Elderly neighbors	10 years 3 years	I help out in the neighborhood, but I don't take on no long jibbity things 'cause between her (wife) and her mother, they come first. But I try to help senior citizens.
Larry Wilson		Wife Mercedes	4 years	It was my choice to be the primary caregiver. I was her husband. I made sure she was taken care of by me. I didn't want her to go in any nursing home (crying).

The Interviews

Private interviews were conducted with each respondent in his home; three respondents preferred to come to the interviewer's home, and one respondent requested to be interviewed at his place of work. Each complete interview included two sessions, with both sessions conducted at the convenience of the respondent. The first interview session focused on the respondent's demographics and his narrative of caregiving, including the number of years he provided care to the care recipient, the nature of the care recipient's illness, the best and worst things about caregiving, and an assessment of relationships among family members in general and specifically in regard to caregiving. The second interview session focused more specifically on the caregiver, including his beliefs, values, the support he received (or did not receive) from others, and his perceived strengths and weaknesses regarding the caregiving role. We note that all questions were followed with tailor-made probes and follow-up questions until no new information emerged. If an interviewer was uncertain about the meaning of a respondent's answer, the interviewer elicited explication with additional questions, such as "Did you mean . . . ?" or, "I'm not sure I understand what you mean, can you explain . . ." and other probes that seemed appropriate to the question and the respondent's initial answer.

Data Analysis

The general approach to data analysis for this project used methods of qualitative research rooted in such fields as anthropology, social work, and religious studies (Black & Rubinstein, 2004; Rubinstein, 1992; Thomas, Groce, & Cooper, 2003). These disciplines have traditions of descriptive analysis in which narrative or story is a major means by which an individual, group, or culture communicates (Geertz, 1973).

In particular, we used the following methods of analyzing qualitative research (Mischler, 1986): After transcription by a dedicated professional transcriptionist, the authors read each transcript carefully, asking, "What, in general, are in the data?" and "How are data relevant to the topic (the tasks and meaning of caregiving) under study?" The next step was large-level sorting of each transcript, in which we coded for broad themes and topics, such as suffering and generativity, intra- and inter-individually in (Silverman, 2001). We also did fine-grained analyses, in which we coded for subthemes and patterns within respondents' entire transcript. In weekly meetings among authors, one "case study" was chosen to be read and discussed (Flyvbjerg, 2006). We focused on patterns and themes in the chosen case and discussed similarities to and differences from other cases (Reissman, 1993). As new data were transcribed and new ideas and themes emerged, we rechecked transcripts, selectively and universally, from respondents who had already completed an interview, in order to confirm or reject particular themes and add others.

In sum, the data we used in this book emerged from responses to formal interview questions, tailor-made follow-up questions, authors' field notes from interviews and team meetings, and informal conversation with respondents that occurred before and after interviews, or when telephoning a respondent to schedule an interview.

As mentioned in the Preface, the major question of our research and this book was: What is the experience of being an elder African-American male caregiver? Our book answers this question in the men's own words.

The content of each chapter explored a theme that all of the men revealed in their narratives. Some themes emerged "naturally." For example, Chapter Two, which explored identity in caregiving, revealed that men's sense of themselves emerged in caregiving but was developed earlier in life and continued to develop and grow through caregiving. In Chapter Four, which examined experiences of suffering in caregiving, men discussed suffering in unique, contextual ways related to being an African-American man. The themes highlighted in each chapter were linked; the linkages are examined throughout the book. Next, we offer a short summary of the book's following chapters.

SUMMARY OF CHAPTERS

Chapter Two: Identity in Caregiving

In this chapter we explored, in men's own words, how each man's caregiving style reflected the person he perceived himself to be. We also examined if and how the legacy of his culture and family prepared him for the role of caregiver. Witnessing and taking part in caregiving earlier in life supported men's belief in the moral worth of both affective and instrumental acts of care for others. The self-worth men found in caregiving reflected and paralleled the self-esteem they found in maintaining important personal values, such as compassion, loyalty, helpfulness to others, and religious or spiritual faith (Mattis et al., 2001).

Chapter Three: Caregiving and Generativity

African-American men revealed a unique type of generativity. It was rooted in their experiences as African-American men, including the foundation of caregiving they received from family, and the experiences of marginalization and racism in the wider world. They believed they had received a legacy from ancestors which was "a responsibility, a warning, and a promise to the 'five generations' that follow them" (Black, Groce, & Harmon, 2011:3). We explored the contextual nature of generativity that men disclosed. That is, their generativity sprang from the unique circumstances of their lives as African Americans; their ability to be generative "despite the small container the larger world allowed them" (Harmon as cited in Black et al., 2011:168).

Chapter Four: Experiences of Suffering

In prior research, elders and caregivers recounted experiences of suffering as a rupture of themselves as whole persons, thus a brokenness in body, mind, and spirit. Persons interviewed stated that their ethnicity, personal biography, cohort history, and current state of mental and physical health were integral to their experience and expression of suffering. Likewise, the context of suffering—in what time of life it occurred, its cause, and its resolution or end—was also taken into account in definitions and descriptions of suffering. In this chapter we asked our caregiving respondents about experiences of suffering in caregiving. We welcomed their general definitions of suffering and asked them to give examples of the experience in their own lives.

Chapter Five: The Strategies of Coping in Caregiving

If an experience is distressful enough to be called suffering, does it ever truly end, or does a residue of the experience continue to assault the wholeness of the person? In this chapter, we explored men's notions of resolving suffering or how they fortified themselves against suffering despite distress. We offered three themes: (1) having goals, (2) the power of the family story, and (3) African-American men's friendship. The themes were often interrelated in men's accounts. Men interviewed for this research revealed the value these themes represented, particularly during caregiving (Black, 2015; Mattis et al., 2001). This chapter also showed older African-American male caregivers to be involved in crucial, reciprocal friendships with other men, which one man described as "what keeps me going."

Chapter Six: African-American Men's Belief Systems

"A book about caregiving can't be written," one of our caregivers said, "without some discussion of our spiritual life." Our caregiving respondents noted the importance of their religious and spiritual beliefs as a means for coping with the daily stress of caregiving. Men's faith offered guidelines for the morality or "rightness" of caregiving. Prayer was a vehicle to speak with God when in distress but also for the purpose of having a relationship with God. For the most part, men believed that God, Allah, or a Higher Power ultimately controlled the precariousness of the caregiving situation. Religious services and fellow members often provided camaraderie and sometimes respite. Men's faith became an internal well in which they laid conflicting emotions to rest and drew a supply of strength and peace.

Chapter Seven: Caregiving as Pilgrimage

In this chapter, a spousal caregiver who had cared for his wife for over 25 years discussed the journey of caregiving as a pilgrimage that the couple traveled together along with family and community. Through the years of being cared for, she incurred other serious illnesses and became increasingly impaired. At the same time, the caregiver's health also waned due to age and illness.

Chapter Eight: Addressing the Silence: African-American Men and Caregiving

As men discussed their care work in the forum of our research, the role of the elder African-American male caregiver was elucidated. Open-ended interview questions prompted discussion of the push and pull of labor-intensive caregiving chores with a well-remembered past and an uncertain future. In many ways, the interview process used in this study promoted a caregiving review, particularly about crucial moments in caregiving. In the lives of elder caregiving men, the meaning of caregiving sometimes became an examination of the self, and a symbol for the meaning and purpose of life.

CHAPTER 2

Identity in Caregiving

PERSONAL IDENTITY

There are multiple theories about identity development and the ways in which personal identity is formed (Erikson, 1963; Mead, 1934). One is the way in which a person perceives himself. This perception occurs through interaction with others and viewing oneself through others' eyes. Through self-perception and the mirroring of others an individual may hold a global description of himself, such as "I am a hard working person," which refers to his approach to all aspects of labor. He may view himself as possessing a fundamental trait that is represented by a value that defines him and is articulated by a recurrent theme (Phillipson & Biggs, 1998), such as "The most important thing is keeping your word. If you say you're going to do something, do it." A sense of continuity in identity over time crystallizes its distinctive features. Also, personal identity integrates new roles throughout the life course. There are descriptions of identity that are dependent on roles, such as "I am a good mechanic" or "I am a loyal church elder." Roles also are contextual and may refer to a particular place and time in life, such as "I was a fair student," or "I am a devoted caregiver." As an individual grows older, he may integrate his self-perception, the discernment of others, and life roles into a macro self-description, for example, "I always try to help anybody who needs help." This description reveals that an identity, whether perceived by self or another, is more than the sum of characteristics, interactions, roles, or self-descriptions (Luborsky, 1993). It is an imprecise structure that takes and changes shape through the experiences of a lifetime.

Identity accommodates its own transformation due to conversion or trauma and the ongoing development of the human person (Brandstadter & Greave, 1994; Janoff-Bulman & Carnes, 2013). Life passages, such as marriage and parenthood, as well as the crises that a person endures, such as illness, disablement, and loss, from childhood to older age, reshape identity (Schroots & Birren, 2002; Sneed & Whitbourne, 2003). Thus, the formation of identity is never completed but remains fluid, being constructed and reconstructed within the contexts of an individual's personal experience and historical biography over time.

ETHNIC IDENTITY

An individual's commitments, such as to a religion, cultural or ethnic group, or organization, are frameworks for a collective identity (Abrams, 1992; Adler, 2012). All men interviewed for this book shared an ethnic identity. Each man's uniqueness as an individual entwined with his communal identity as an African-American man born in the first half of the 20th century, and his lifelong, positive and negative experiences. Cultural and social rules, tacit and overt, were bequeathed from men's smaller and larger worlds (Hines & Boyd-Franklin, 1996). The men's smaller world (family, community) handed down advice about interacting with the dominant society. Advice often came as a warning about how to maneuver carefully through life. From the larger world (public life, society) came similar warnings to African-American men, but for a different purpose—submission. The disparate objectives for these warnings created a tension within African-American men named by Du Bois (1903b) as a "double consciousness." One perception that men held of themselves was cultivated by family. It portrayed a man as confident, responsible, and capable of leading his own ship and defending it. Another portrait emerged through the eyes of the dominant society—as the "other." Lesser jobs with lesser pay, limitations in housing options and education, and implicit and explicit laws that demanded subservience in the larger world, mocked African-American men's masculinities (David, 2013; Mutua, 2006; Pierre et al., 2001). The uncanny experience of "being of two minds" shaped African-American men's identity from childhood through adulthood (Courtenay, 2000).

The men also shared a cohort identity due to their place in time and historical background. Cognizant that the American Dream had a different meaning for people of color, African-American men discerned that their major resources in life were people, particularly family and especially older African-American men—relatives or nonrelatives—who modeled a way to succeed within a limited sphere of options. One caregiving respondent described how this occurred at his job in the US post office. The men who went before him, such as fathers, uncles, or neighbors, held excellent credentials for the job of mentor.

> In the post office I got closer to guys who were older and some were Second World War vets. And they were talking about the racism and poverty they experienced during the war, and still, in the 1950s. And I gravitated to them because of wanting to learn. Now I was depressed in there because all whites was in charge and the blacks was the laborers. And we couldn't break that barrier.

As mentioned earlier, African-American men had served in segregated armed forces during World War II with the belief that their second-class status would be upgraded due to their service. In wake of overt discrimination during and after the war, men realized that racism had been threaded into the political and social ethos of society. In a counter-offensive, many African-American men overtly assumed their racial identity; they acknowledged ancient African-American traditions, recalled their distant and recent history, and applauded their differences from the dominant culture (Groce, 2002). They also honed bonds of family and kinship; bolstered group identity; and capitalized on their adaptive strengths to reform the structure of a society that ignored, shamed, or penalized them (Baldwin, 1961).

Both despite and because of the cultural and social changes occurring throughout the United States when African-American men were coming of age, that is, in the 1940s and 1950s, violence became an aspect of social protest. Unpredictability lay at the core of how men's lives might unfold in this environment. This unpredictability required, on the part of African-American men, (1) a learned response of control over self and circumstances and (2) circumspect interactions with the larger society. The men in our study believed that the tension of double consciousness, the history of adapting their strengths to hardships, the need for role flexibility in supporting a family, and guarding personal identities from the wider world, reflected their distant past, steered the future, and augured their success as men and as caregivers (Moore, 2010).

THE DISTANT PAST

Memory is critical in the lives of marginalized peoples (Climo & Cattell, 2002). A crucial aspect of the communal identity of oppression was to nourish memories and bestow them to future generations. Collective memory recalled ancestors divided by slavery; the young and strong could be kept or sold; the old and ill were dispensable (Raboteau, 1978). The end of slavery brought a new form of economic slavery through sharecropping, which conferred ongoing family dissolution. Migration from southern states to the north for work often meant leaving loved ones and land and the strong sense of connection with place, which is an anchor for identity.

The African-American men we interviewed revealed the deleterious ways that racism in the distant and recent past—in access to education and opportunities for social mobility—can influence the present—in socioeconomic disproportion, health disparities, and a decreased life span—even when personal assets, such as intelligence, good health, or subjective well-being seemed capable of overcoming inequities (David, 2013). The effect of traumatic events that occurred in a group's communal history on present worldview is significant in the construction of group memory *and* identity (Kidron, 2003).

Relating the communal history of African Americans to family caregiving, one caregiver told us, "We didn't have the economic resources and we didn't trust the system. We depended on each other." Home caregiving provided safety for a loved one (Hopp & Thomas, 2014). It also supported a belief in the moral obligation of reciprocal caregiving (Brodaty & Donkin, 2009; Hamilton & Sandelowski, 2004). Did the legacy of men's cultural tradition prepare him for his role as caregiver?

Many African-American male caregivers perceived that an assessment of their caregiving was two-fold. Internally, each caregiver monitored his own behavior—what he had done well or poorly was measured against the care recipient's health, cognition, or mood. Externally, he was aware that the smaller world of family and other intimates bolstered his venture in caregiving; his caregiving identity was enhanced by their support (Hasselkus & Murray, 2007; Lane & King, 2012). Some men in the study noted that the wider, White world also was observing their caregiving behaviors.

In this chapter, we explore how each man's caregiving actions reflected his identity or the person he perceived himself (and desired) to be. A man's caregiving identity was revealed in a number of ways. Among them were (1) his agreement to be interviewed; (2) the caregiving experiences he disclosed; and (3) the answers he gave to interview questions, such as, How had he come to be his loved one's primary caregiver? Had he given care to more than one person in his life? Did he think of himself as a caregiver? We note that several men in our study, although having given care for many years, did not see themselves as a caregiver. Perhaps significant to a man's response to the question of whether he thought of himself as a caregiver was how he interpreted the word—was it a positive or negative term? Also key to each man's caregiving identity was how he appraised his motives, intentions, and acts within the caregiving role, and if and how others took note of his role as a caregiver (Tise, 2015).

MR. EDDIE GILMORE

We begin our exploration of identity in caregiving by introducing Mr. Eddie Gilmore, aged 64, who was interviewed in his West Philadelphia home. Mr. Gilmore is of average height and keeps the physique of an athlete due to regularly playing tennis, a regimen of exercise, and an active schedule. At the time of the interview, he was also remodeling his home.

Mr. Gilmore has been the primary caregiver for his wife, Donna, for 10 years. He began caregiving after she suffered the effects of two strokes during a medical procedure to correct an irregular heart rhythm. At first, he used accrued leave time from his supervisory position at the post office.

> When they (the strokes) happened, I took leave. My decision at that time was to go back to work. When she was discharged, we had to do outpatient therapy. And that lasted 4 months. So I took it month by month to see how her condition was. After a year passed I saw it was going to be long term and she needed my care 24/7 and I retired.

The Gilmores have been married 41 years and have two daughters. Although Mr. Gilmore described his wife as "the picture of health," the strokes rendered her aphasic, which is an inability to produce and understand speech, and usually results from brain damage caused by injury or disease. Mr. Gilmore described his wife's difficulty in talking with others as "suffering" due to the depth of her frustration that she was unable to give voice to her thoughts.

Mr. Gilmore's approach to caregiving would be described as all-encompassing. He oversees every aspect of his wife's care and named himself her "lifeline." When asked to describe a typical day of caregiving, he replied,

> I live two lives. Most people start caregiving in the morning. I'm up half the night watching her breathe 'cause she has sleep apnea. I know you can die from it. She wakes up suddenly and her heart is playing catch up. That's how the irregular heartbeat started. I listen to her in the morning and make sure I don't hear anything out of the ordinary as far as slurred speech. I'm always checking to see she maintains her weight, has proper meals, and takes her medicine. Grooming is a factor; I make sure of that, too.

Mr. Gilmore considered caregiving a legacy from his family of origin. When asked if he had witnessed caregiving in his home or community while growing up, he replied:

> When you grow up in the 50s which is when I was born, in the Afro- American household that's a given. As your grandmother got older, or if you were fortunate enough to have a great-grandmother, you were committed to making sure she was cared for. At that time, it wasn't so much sickness, it was aging—that was the terminology. When I was coming up, it was built in. If you were 15, 16, 17, you took care of grandma.

Mr. Gilmore was born and raised in North Carolina and came to Philadelphia in 1971 after serving in the Vietnam War. He grew up in an era—the 1950s—when after-school chores included hands-on care for elder relatives or simply spending time with them. According to Mr. Gilmore, values such as respect for the aged, consistent interaction with them, and their participation in all aspects of family life were "built in," as was his "work ethic." He continued to describe a "typical" day.

> I move from the time I get up in the morning until I go to bed. The folks that know me want to know where I get all the energy from. I tell them as far as I can think back, work ethic is learned at home. I remember at 5 years old I was carrying papers. It was something that grew up in me and it's still in me.

Mr. Gilmore revealed how he saw himself—as a hard worker—throughout his narrative. The roles he assumed in the past—daily interaction with his grandmother, responsibility for a paper route at age 5—foreshadowed the intense labor that he put into caregiving.

Mr. Gilmore acknowledged that caregiving does not take place in a vacuum. He reported that he is "always on guard." For him, caregiving included protecting his wife from the "good intentions" of extended family members who see Donna irregularly and remember her as she was before the stroke.

> We was at a wedding 2 months ago. I'm sitting there with Donna, which I always do because I'm very protective of her. One of her first cousins, Carol, comes over and she gets real close, she is right on top of her. I'm like, "Carol, Carol" (waves his hand) because they don't realize. "Aunt Donna, how you doing, Aunt Donna?" (Loud voice) I say, "Carol, remember Donna is still in therapy." She says, "Oh." 'Cause she's going on and on about what happened 40, 50 years ago. Donna is thinking, but she can't say what she's thinking. When they grew up together, I wasn't there so I can't express nothing.

Mr. Gilmore explained that family and friends commend his caregiving. And although Donna's relatives praise his devotion to her, it is difficult for them to comprehend the physical *and* emotional effects aphasia has on his wife. He mentioned that the wider, White world also takes note of how he cares for Donna.

> When I'm around Caucasians or Asians, which I am weekly because I take her to rehab and the speech therapists and those in the hierarchy are Caucasians. But the classroom setting (clients) is 75% Black. They all look at me as strength. They say, "You stood up as an Afro-American male and you are an inspiration for everybody in the group." I told them, "It's there—Black men are taking care of their spouses." But maybe more so with the older males because when you are talking about young folks—(pause). When I was coming up, it was built in.

Mr. Gilmore's themes of inheriting an ethic of hard work and giving physical and emotional care to loved ones linked his story of caregiving with his life story. He reported that his natural talents were sharpened through suffering. In a later chapter, we will see how he used his role as a soldier in Vietnam to further hone his identity.

MR. JAMES KELCH

We introduce Mr. James Kelch, a 76-year-old, well-dressed, well-spoken widower who lived in the Wynnefield section of the city and preferred to be interviewed in the interviewer's home. Mr. Kelch had been the primary caregiver for his wife, Beverly, for over 5 years and had been married 38 years at the time of her death. Mr. Kelch, a social work professor, was retired and lived alone in the home the couple shared with their three children. When Mr. Kelch was asked whether he witnessed caregiving while growing up, he replied: "My grandparents lived with us and my mother did a lot in taking care of them so I was knowledgeable about the role, but I didn't really participate." He explained:

> I always thought it was a feminine role, that caregivers are women. This is what women did. They have the gentle touch for bathing and taking care of patients. I never imagined that I would be doing this. I never saw myself in that role until I was in it (laughs).

Mr. Kelch brought up a salient issue in research on male caregivers in general—men are second-string replacements for tasks that female caregivers perform, from emotional support to cleaning after incontinence. Yet research has shown that almost 4 out of 10 caregivers are men (NAC & AARP, 2015; Russell, 2007; Scharlach, 2008). As Mr. Kelch came to realize through caregiving, gender identity is fluid, and gendered roles can be changed by context, for example, through illness, economics, or living arrangements. When asked, Mr. Kelch described the first signs of his wife's illness.

> Her weight loss was alarming. She became very weak and it was hard for her to function. That was the first sign we were in trouble. The doctor gave her a number of tests and found out she was not absorbing food. There were complications, and her autoimmune system was compromised. They tried various diets and then the feeding tube was placed in.

When asked how he came to be her primary caregiver, he responded:

> Our oldest daughter was married, so she was off with her husband. Our son was in college at Virginia Union. Our youngest daughter was in high school. Until she went to the university, she was with me and helped with her mom. But when she went to school—she didn't want to go and I convinced her that I would be there to pick up what her mother needed. I just eventually became the caregiver.

Mr. Kelch described a scenario that was typical for our respondents. They encouraged their children to acquire an education and career, which sometimes meant the children moved out of state. Although they may have wanted to help their fathers, and the men may have needed their help, the children "were living their own lives." Mr. Kelch continued, "So, then, Beverly was there helpless and I was the only one to do it . . . and then I had to play it to the best of my ability." His comment hinted that, at first, caregiving was a role he "fell into."

When asked, Mr. Kelch described himself as a "caregiver." The interviewer commented on the fact that some men *do not* describe themselves as caregivers despite the breadth of their tasks. Mr. Kelch looked surprised. "What do they call themselves? Oh, yes, I was a caregiver. It's an active, not a passive role." He talked about the least favorite activity of caregiving: "The potty. That was always rough because I would have the retching reaction and you know I'd have to wipe her. That was rough, that was rough."

Mr. Kelch, in middle age, assumed the role of primary caregiver for his wife and reframed his picture of "who" a caregiver is. The necessity *and* desire to care for his wife in their home superseded Mr. Kelch's belief that caregiving was a "woman's" role. During the interview, he recalled his years of caregiving with wonder.

> I am sometimes in awe of my own experience. I look back and say, "Did I do that?" How was I able to do all I did? I don't know. I don't know if you [had] proposed that beforehand, that I could say, "Yes, I will do that." But I did. What needed to be done I did.

Mr. Kelch's response to his caregiving accomplishments mirrored men's surprise at being able to carry out certain tasks, such as those that surrounded incontinence and the last stages of dementia, when loved ones no longer recognized them. Although Mr. Kelch said he would "do it all again," he retrospectively realized he had not known the depth of strength he needed to assume the role of caregiver.

During our interview, Mr. Kelch scrutinized past decisions he believed had shaped him. Earlier in life he rejected a role his father handed down—"authority figure."

> In growing up I wanted to be a good provider, but I wanted to be more than that. I wanted to know my children and operate on them as a friend as well as a father. My father never wanted to get friendly with me or chummy. He wanted clear lines of authority. I wanted to break that down [with my children].

When asked how he had changed the "father" role with his children, Mr. Kelch addressed what it was like to be an African-American father.

> I think you're always concerned about your children, always hoping for the best, but fearing for the worst. But I didn't let the weight of the oppression that African Americans lived under, and that I felt was on me, fall on my children. I tried to protect them. I wanted them to have a sense that they were capable of anything.

Mr. Kelch took the legacy of ethnic and gender beliefs that were passed down to him—that only women are caregivers, that fathers are authority figures, and that African Americans inherit a sense of oppression that fall to their children—and rescripted it for his children. He fostered a warm connection with them, provided them with an excellent education, and assured them that their goals were within reach. When his wife became ill, he altered his ideas about "men's work" to include hands-on caregiving. We will return to Mr. Kelch in later chapters.

MR. FRED PARKER

Mr. Parker, a 76-year-old African-American man, was born and raised in South Philadelphia. He worked as a mechanic and preferred to be interviewed at his place of work. He was of average height and weight and appeared to be in excellent physical condition. Although he described his emotional health as "excellent," he described his physical health as "fair" due to diabetes. Mr. Parker was a United States veteran and a former semi-professional baseball player. His friends described him as a "leader."

Mr. Parker gave primary care to his first wife. When the interviewer asked him about the first signs of her illness, he replied:

> She started spitting up blood. We went to the doctors and they did X-rays and ultrasounds and found out she had a tumor on her lung. Then they did a biopsy and found out it was cancerous. We went through all the treatments—the chemo, radiation, all that stuff. But it was unrepairable because once they did the radiation it broke the cancer up and spread it to different parts of her body.

Mr. Parker said he had not seen caregiving in his home, except for the care that his parents gave "to us children." When asked how long he had cared for his wife, Mr. Parker replied:

> Her episode with cancer was 6 years. But the first 4 years she was functional. She was able to get around and do for herself. When it moved from her lungs to her brain is when she became bedridden. She couldn't move, but she would have good days and bad days.

When asked how he came to be his wife's primary caregiver, he said that his wife requested he take care of her; she did not want "outside people coming in."

> I told her, "I'll do whatever you want." She made me promise not to leave her in the hospital. The day before she died I had to take her to the hospital to get catheterized to move her urine. In the hospital they said, "Oh, no, she's here to stay." I said, "No, when you people get done what you're doing I'm taking my wife home." They said, "You can't do that." I said, "Lady, move out of my way." I picked her up, carried her out, put her in the car, and took her home.

Mr. Parker said that one of the most difficult situations during his wife's illness was "dealing with the doctors." Because the couple knew Mrs. Parker's illness was terminal, she wanted to visit as many family members as possible. Many of them lived out of state.

Mr. Parker: They (doctors) were like "You can't do this . . . you can't do that . . . you got to lay down." My wife wanted to get out and visit people and see aunts and uncles and cousins. We knew the bottom line because they had given her a year to live and she wanted to move around. We told the doctors, "We are going to Cleveland" or "We are going to California." "Oh, you can't do that. You can't move her." I would ask, "Why?" This is what she wanted to do. We already knew the bottom line, so why are you restricting us?

Interviewer: So, did you go?

Mr. Parker: Oh yeah, yeah, yeah. We went everywhere she wanted to go and every time we would come back the doctors would say, "Oh wow, she's doing great. You should take her . . ." We'd say, "We are; we're going again." When it got down to the final week my wife said, "Look, I don't want to die in the hospital. I want to die at home with my family." She said, "You got to promise me that you won't leave me there" (crying). I said, "Okay."

Interviewer: Take your time

Mr. Parker: (continuing to cry)

Interviewer: It sounds like you had a tremendous relationship.

Mr. Parker: Oh, she was a sweetheart. The love of my life.

When Mr. Parker was asked if he considered himself his wife's caregiver, he replied, "Not really, no." He described himself as "a needed husband doing what needed to be done." He revealed that after his wife's death, he realized his caregiving duties were not over.

> Just after my wife passed my mother got sick. I brought her down from New York, and it was almost the same pattern. But my mother didn't have cancer; she was just up in age. She couldn't function for herself. It was Old Timer's. Then Alzheimer's came on and evolved, and it ended up I was [doing] breakfast, lunch, and dinner, bedtime, bathing. You know, the whole process. And with my mom I felt this was the least I could do because she took care of me when I couldn't do it.

Mr. Parker described the caregiving he gave to his wife and mother as a natural part of life. He gave little thought to assuming the roles *and* identity of "needed" husband and son. He added, "For any of my family, if this is what I have to do, then it's what I do." We will return to Mr. Parker in later chapters.

MR. HORACE BRUNSON

We continue with Mr. Horace Brunson, who was interviewed in the interviewer's home. Mr. Brunson, a 70-year-old man of average height and weight, appeared years younger. When asked about his health, Mr. Brunson reported that he visits his doctor every 6 months. "It's good. He (doctor) checks me out and everything is good so far, thank God for that." Despite an arthritic knee, he continues to ride a motorcycle, a pastime he enjoyed since youth. With a smile, he repeated how his niece described him. "My Uncle Horace is 70 years old but he ain't like them old 70s. He's a young 70." Similar to Mr. Parker, Mr. Brunson continued to work every day as a driver for a local insurance company.

Mr. Brunson was married and widowed twice and became the primary caregiver for both wives when they became ill. His first wife was Mattie, with whom he had three children. Mattie's symptoms appeared when they were on a vacation cruise.

> When we came back, we went to the doctor and discovered her blood count was low. She went in the hospital right away. She needed blood, but she was scared to take it from the hospital because that's how Arthur Ashe got AIDS. So me and my three kids went to the hospital to see if our blood matched up, but it didn't.

Mr. Brunson and their children hoped they could donate *their* blood for her transfusion and allay Mattie's fears. This family portrait illustrated the emotional *and* physical support they gave to Mattie. Mr. Brunson continued.

> She had colon cancer and it was real bad. This was 1994. They kept her for 2 weeks after two operations. They took a lot of stuff out of her. At first she didn't want chemo or radiation. She came home for about 4 months, then this knot came back in her. She went for chemo and they found she had jaundice; she had septic [sepsis], and from that day she was going downhill.

Mr. Brunson's plain-spoken manner highlights the starkness of Mattie's diagnosis and illness. He described the last year of her life.

> It was a slow process. She needed fluid. She'd go to the hospital and come home. Then she decided to sleep downstairs. I made me a little thing on the floor and I slept next to her. Then she went back in the hospital. There was nobody in the room with her, so I asked the nurse if I could stay. After work I'd spend the night and get up and do for her instead of calling the nurse. I helped them [nurses] out as much as I could. Then she got someone in her room so I couldn't stay, but I went every day. I never missed a day. I would go to work, go to the hospital. That was my job.

Several of the caregiving men, similar to Mr. Brunson, undertook the responsibility of caregiving as they would a job or career. Some men learned new duties in the role of caregiver, such as cooking and keeping house, and became proud of their skills. They brought together the feminine qualities of nurturance with a masculine desire to be proficient at instrumental tasks. This blend of characteristics revealed competency as both a man and a caregiver and often provided satisfaction despite caregiving distress (Black et al., 2008). In Mr. Brunson's case, the affective tasks of caregiving, such as sleeping at the hospital and "never missing a day," granted insight into his dedication to both his wife and what he perceived as his "work." "So, this was the part I had to deal with and I didn't have a problem with it because I loved her and I enjoyed doing it for her."

Mr. Brunson reported that he had not witnessed caregiving in his family of origin. His grandparents died before he was born, and his parents were healthy until their deaths. A legacy he *had* inherited from his family, which he repeated throughout the interview, was the importance of keeping your word. It was a core aspect of Mr. Brunson's identity.

> When I tell somebody something, I want to live to that fully. The one thing I do despise is liars. My parents raised me if you say you are going to do something, let your word be your bond. If you can't do it, pick up the phone and say I can't do it. But don't lie. That's what I loved about both my wives. They was good ladies. When they said they was going to do something, you didn't have to worry about it. It was done.

For Mr. Brunson, marriage was a commitment that fell under the rubric of keeping your word. "I was there for Mattie as much as possible because I feel like they say when you are married you are married until death will you part." After Mattie's death, working at the insurance company and assisting neighbors with house and lawn chores helped him endure the loss.

> I was telling my daughter this morning that I don't have no grief over her mother (Mattie) anymore, and this August it will be 19 years that she's gone. See, Barbara (second wife) helped me get through [the death of] my first wife by being with me and going places [together].

Barbara, Mr. Brunson's second wife, had been his neighbor. After Mattie's death, he noticed that "Barbara could use some help" with household tasks. Her health problems had begun long before their marriage.

> Barbara knew I loved my first wife. But with Barbara, the way she went about things made me really like her a lot and begin to fall in love. A long time before we got married I would do things like cut her hedges. See, even then she was sick and couldn't do a lot. I did lots of vacuuming, clean the windows. She didn't have to worry about no snow in her front yard.

When asked about the nature of Barbara's illness, Mr. Brunson replied, "It started with her breathing, you know shortness of breath." Only the constant use of oxygen relieved Barbara's symptoms. Mr. Brunson estimated that he was her primary caregiver for 6 years.

> Her lungs I guess were kind of messed up. And it got to the place that she needed more oxygen, more units. It was kind of a long road with her because you know she's been around for a while with that oxygen. She told me, "Horace, every time I go to the hospital, I go lower and lower. There's no help."

Mr. Brunson said that, similar to how he cared for Mattie during her illness, "It wasn't no problem to help Barbara with whatever she wanted."

> Like during the night she would say, "Horace, can you go downstairs and check my oxygen" "No problem." This after working all day. "Can you get me this? Can you get me that? Can you stop by the drugstore?" "No problem." 'Cause that was my job to make sure whatever she needed, I do for her and I had no problem with it.

At the time of the interview, it had been a year since Barbara passed. Mr. Brunson realized that although he continued to mourn her, he also recognized what helped him manage his grief.

> Now I'm grieving over Barbara. Like yesterday on my way home from work I was crying a little bit. But I am so glad I am still working. The more busy I am... When I'm around people I talk, my mind don't have to be on it (Barbara's death) as much. Work for me is therapy.

Viewing caregiving as work and naming work as therapy offered a window into Mr. Brunson's mindset. Work was a necessity for Mr. Brunson not solely to earn money but also to keep busy, and to socialize with others. Working productively as a caregiver, at his job, or for his neighbors helped him cope with his wives' illnesses and deaths.

Mr. Brunson shared two recent conversations. One occurred while Barbara was still alive and receiving breathing treatments. He and a therapist discussed caregiving tasks when she visited their home.

> I was talking to this lady who came to give Barbara some instrument for her breathing and I was telling her about my first dying (first wife Mattie's death) and going through the illness with Barbara. She said, "God bless you because a lot of people can't even take care of one person." See, a lot of people cannot deal with sickness. They are ready to walk out the door when somebody get ill. But for me it's so easy because I enjoy taking care of that person because I love that person. Because unless somebody's got a good heart, it's hard to really understand what being a caregiver means.

Mr. Brunson described Mattie's death as "my first dying." The minimalism of his language communicated that he did not fight against Mattie's dying but endured it with her and journeyed with her to her death. The second conversation occurred with one of Horace's buddies.

> I got a friend in South Carolina. He told me, "Horace, I wish I was a guy like you 'cause I was a woman chaser." (Pause) That was never in my world, never. Give me one good lady. That's all I want, one good lady and I will focus on her.

Mr. Brunson remained committed to a principle of honesty that is both complex and narrow in that it leaves little "wiggle" room. It provided him with a fixed compass for how to behave in every situation: Keep your word, love one lady at a time without counting the cost, when death comes mourn deeply, and in the present stay busy and focus on what is in front of you. We will revisit Mr. Brunson in a later chapter, as he speaks about suffering, mourning, and coping with the afterward of spousal loss.

MR. HARRY STOKES

Mr. Harry Stokes, aged 83, was a tall, distinguished-looking man who carried himself with confidence. He was described with a smile by another respondent as "the picture of sartorial splendor." Mr. Stokes lived with his wife in a large, beautifully manicured home just outside the city. Another respondent said of Mr. Stokes: "You see how neat he keeps himself? His home looks the same way."

Mr. Stokes mentioned several careers he enjoyed, often holding down two jobs at the same time. He had been a basketball official, bartender, social worker, and eventually retired from the personnel department of the federal government. Mr. Stokes cared for his mother for over 15 years until her death at age 95. When asked about the nature of her illness, he replied, "Rheumatoid arthritis. See, she was a day's worker and in those days when you did day's work you didn't mop nothing. You got down on your knees and scrubbed." Mr. Stokes recalled first noticing his mother's debility.

> She was having difficulty getting up and standing and negotiating steps. And when they did the X-rays, they discovered all the cartilage in both her knees was gone. She was able to move around a little. Then when she was in her late 70s, early 80s, she had a mastectomy. But she never got radiation or chemo. She was clear. So the cancer didn't make the arthritis worse, but it was another illness, and she needed more help.

When asked how he came to be her primary caregiver, Mr. Stokes said, "I was the only one. I didn't have any siblings; she was widowed and, ahh, I did what I had to do." He described his daily caregiving routine. "I'd get up in the mornings; she was living over on North Bernard Street off Westminster Avenue. I'd stop before I go to work and fix her breakfast. Then I'd fix up a little lunch. She had a refrigerator up in her room."

Mr. Stokes's comment "I did what I had to do" highlighted an important theme in men's narratives of caregiving. When a loved one became disabled, they considered it *their* responsibility to take on the role of caregiver. Although his mother's sister stayed with his mother during the day, he was reluctant to put "a lot of pressure" on his elderly aunt. He continued:

> After work, I'd go by and fix her evening meal. Then I'd go to my second job. You know what people used to say to me? "You gonna retire soon?" I said, "Well, it's like everything else. God gives you the strength to serve and you are put here to do just that."

When asked about his mother's personality, Mr. Stokes laughed.

> Oh, she was sharp and feisty, and she was real old school. She was also very, very smart and didn't have a formal education. She had what we call motherwit.

When asked whether, during this time, he thought of himself as his mother's caregiver, Mr. Stokes shook his head:

> I didn't see myself as a caregiver. I saw myself as the son that's supposed to do what he's supposed to do for his mother. Because caregiver to me, maybe it's just me, but if I say I was the caregiver for my mother it's like, "Well, I don't want to be a caregiver but I have to be. It's a job." No, I was her son; she was my mother.

Mr. Stokes believed that the label of "caregiver" made caregiving seem obligatory—a role that someone could not refuse. Instead, he reported that he was "honored" to have cared for his mother. He also learned to have respect for the dead from his mother's diligence in visiting those who mourn.

> I tell people this story a lot of times—My mother and I'd be walking up the street and if we get near a funeral home in the neighborhood, and if there was crepe on the door, she'd say, "You stand right there. I'm going in and see if it's anybody I know." And she'd go in. In those days they didn't have it in the newspaper.

Mr. Stokes and the interviewer laughed, and the interviewer commented, "Well, every time there's a funeral in West Philly for somebody we know, I know we'll see Harry Stokes there." Mr. Stokes answered. "Absolutely I will be there. It just comes natural to me."

When Mr. Stokes was asked what it means to be an African-American older man who has given care to another person, he thought for a moment, searching for the right words.

> I would have to say I was fortunate. I was able to get an insight on what it's like when you watch a person get old. It's an education. You hear about these things, but now you're experiencing it first-hand. So what does it mean? It means to me that I'm prepared to assist anybody that is going through something like this. I will assist you in any way because I know what it involves, what it takes. I guess I have that sensitivity I never realized I had, because of going through what I went through.

Mr. Stokes's thoughtful response revealed that perhaps persons glean from their experiences what they already hold inside. Caregiving was an education for Mr. Stokes because he was open to learning about the varied aspects of old age that emerged during his mother's long life. He navigated his life course with the same moral scope that guided his mother's journey. We will return to Mr. Stokes in a later chapter.

MR. ELLIS MOORE

Another respondent for whom caregiving became an education was Mr. Ellis Moore. Mr. Moore, 76 years old, was a tall, distinguished-looking widower who preferred to be interviewed in the interviewer's home. One respondent described Mr. Moore as ""respected in the sports world and admired in his community. He's a really affable person, not antagonistic at all." Mr. Moore was a basketball player in the Industrial and Government Leagues of Philadelphia. He retired from the post office as a mail-flow mechanic.

When asked, Mr. Moore said that his wife became ill shortly after his retirement. He was her primary caregiver for approximately 6 years.

> She was diagnosed with cancer in '94 or '95. Then it came back in 2000 and went everywhere. They wanted to put her in the hospital but I said, "No, we will do this here." See, when it came back, she was helpless.

When asked how he came to be her primary caregiver, he explained:

> They had some alternatives like a nursing home, but I said she wasn't going in no nursing home, so I made the decision. I said, "I am going to be here." She was thankful, but you know we had our times. It weren't all peaches and cream. But I said, "I am going to be here." She was always telling people, "He can't do that today; he's got to help me" (laughter).

When asked what his wife was like as a person, Mr. Moore shrugged and smiled.

> We were married 40 years. Both of us would say, "I'm leaving." "No, I'm leaving."' But that was all a bunch of talk. It didn't go no further than that. Most everybody liked her but me (laughter).

When asked about the nature of the care he gave to her, Mr. Moore replied:

> I get up in the morning and feed her. That's the first thing in the morning. The nurses come by, I think they got an hour to come over and do something, but they do nothing. I fired I don't know how many of them because they come in and go in the refrigerator. Sometimes the boyfriends [of the care aides] was waiting outside. Finally I said, "Don't send anybody (aides) anymore." So I kind of learned how to cook and she could kind of tell me what to do with the stuff, you know. I ain't never been no cook. She just told me to go to the

> store and get this, get that. A couple of the neighbors, they would stop in every now and then and drop something (food) off. She had to take Codeine and Oxycontin. I was almost a doctor, I thought, the way I was administering the drugs.

Mr. Moore was disappointed with the formal aides sent by healthcare agencies he contacted. Although neighbors were helpful, he worried about taking advantage of their offer to "sit with" his wife. Similar to several of our caregiving men, Mr. Moore retrospectively wondered how he was able to take on the caregiving role. He never imagined it would become part of his "job" as a husband because he had not assumed these tasks in the first six decades of his life. We will return to Mr. Moore in a later chapter.

MR. ELLIOT DAVIS

As we continue our study of identity in caregiving men, we introduce Mr. Elliot Davis, an 87-year-old widower who was the primary caregiver for his wife, Gemma. Like Mr. Kelch and Mr. Brunson, he was also a widower at the time of our interview. Unlike the men introduced previously, Mr. Davis had not received a clear family legacy about caregiving. We explore in this section whether a lack of family legacy in the construction of his identity made a difference in his approach to caregiving.

Mr. Davis' mother was hospitalized when he was 13 years old and, apart from a few brief meetings, he never knew his father. Yet he wove a strong cultural identity as an African-American man based on his mother's hard work, his experiences with the Black Church, and emulating well-known persons he chose as role models. He successfully constructed a personal identity as a sophisticate in the arts, an activist for African Americans, and reached the pinnacle of success within his chosen field of work.

Mr. Davis met the interviewer in the lobby of his apartment building. As they rode the elevator to an upper floor, several tenants from the building entered the elevator. Mr. Davis cheerfully greeted each person. Once inside his studio apartment, the interviewer was invited to sit at a wooden dinette table. When asked to whom or what he attributed his success, Mr. Davis considered. "I think it has to do with the hard knocks that most people go through when they are young." Mr. Davis described growing up in an urban area, the surviving son of a single parent.

> My mother migrated from a small town in Georgia. I never met my only sister; she died of pneumonia when they still lived there. So I grew up in North Philadelphia and came through the Depression years. We moved from apartment to apartment because we couldn't keep up the rent.

Mr. Davis clarified that his passions and successes resulted from mental strength, along with his ability to cultivate solitary outlets because of being on his own at an early age. "My mother was hospitalized when I was a young teen, so I considered myself on my own from that point, doing the best I could with no family or anyone." When asked about his father, he replied with little emotion.

> I briefly knew my father. My mother took me to meet him when I was about 10 years old. (Pause) I went to see him once when I made the track team in high school. I asked for track shoes from the pawn shop. He said, "I don't have any money." I didn't pursue it. Mother was in the hospital and this man, identified as my father, didn't volunteer a little thing like sneakers. He should have been proud. When I hear Billie Holiday's song "God Bless the Child"—"Mother may have, sister may have . . . God bless the child who has his own." That was my theme for the rest of my life. That's what fortified me: *never ever* depend on anyone else (Mr. Davis's emphasis).

The account of his early years provided clues to Mr. Davis's identity. He used the word "fortified" to describe how his past shaped him. His hardships had not embittered him; they had strengthened him. Although Mr. Davis had no mentor to guide him, he relied on the practical and spiritual advice of various African-American church pastors whose sermons he heard. He also chose to model himself on an African-American activist.

> I identified with Paul Robeson and tried to walk in his shoes. He was against racism; he was a practicing attorney and gave that up to start going on tours of all the African-American churches. We supported him because he had no income. They took his passport away because he got involved with Russia. They considered him a Communist. Today "terrorist" is a bad word. Fifty years ago "communist" was the bad word. He was an idol because he sacrificed so much for us, not for himself.

Mr. Davis molded himself into a man with a purpose. His goal, which he achieved, was to rise higher than the obstacles he endured in his young life and to assist young African Americans he met on this path.

When asked about caregiving, Mr. Davis reported that he had been the primary caregiver for his wife, Gemma. He described their meeting at a local factory where they both worked. He depicted the economic and social circumstances of African-American young adults in the 1940s and 1950s.

> We dated and learned we had common interests. She was very intelligent. During that time most of the young men and women didn't go to college because they couldn't afford it; they went to work in industry. There wasn't a lot of opportunities for us.

When asked when and how he became her primary caregiver, he laughed.

> Oh, from practically the beginning of our relationship. One of the things that occurred with her health was female problems. Once a month she'd be down for 3 days. I'd do the washing on a scrub board. I scrubbed my son's diapers. In the beginning of our marriage she was hospitalized at least five times. One of the last operations was a hysterectomy and 6 months later she still had problems.

Mr. Davis explained that Gemma's medical bills forced him to take on two jobs "to keep up with the expenses of her ailments." His caregiving duties became more demanding when she was stricken with several illnesses.

> She got a job in South Philadelphia. I'd pick her up and take her to work. She was taking hormones which contributed to her breast cancer. She had breast surgery and did chemotherapy and went into remission. Then a problem came up with diverticulitis. On top of that she smoked incessantly because of her pressure job. She had emphysema. She was constantly pulling this little oxygen tank. The big tank was in our house. I filled it every day. After a year the cancer came back. They started the chemo again and all the hair came out and we were always looking for wigs. When I took her to the hospital, you couldn't find a wheelchair; I had to rent one and keep it in my car. It got to the point—and I think that's where frustration set in with me. A simple thing became difficult—taking the wheelchair out of the car.

Mr. Davis remarked that frustration often "set in" not with the crises that occurred in caregiving, but with its small, repetitive tasks.

> When we got to the hospital, I'd put her in the wheelchair and park the car. She was annoyed she had to wait for me. After the second-round chemotherapy the doctor said, "There's nothing else we can do." We went to Sloan Kettering and they prescribed radiation. By that time she couldn't do stairs. I put a bathroom and hospital bed in the dining room. Then her veins collapsed; medication had to go into a vein in her heart. Every day I had to flush that and put the medicine in just like a doctor. It got to the point that it was tiring and frustrating. When

> I brought her home from the hospital, I'd park on the sidewalk so she could walk in the house. The pressure was so great, half the time I left my car on the sidewalk. I'd come out and I'd have tickets on the car. I don't know who called [the police]; the car wasn't blocking the street. They see what you go through, but there's no sympathy.

The listener could hear Mr. Davis's annoyance as he recalled these incidents. He received little support from any corner. Although Gemma's sister came one Saturday a month to "help out," Mr. Davis remained on call. He was expected to be available to help his sister-in-law with *her* errands.

> When she (sister-in-law) was ready to leave, I took her food shopping, then home. By the time you come back all hell breaks loose when you walk in the door. "Where were you?" All of that you had to endure. (Pause) See, what she was going through—a lot of bitterness and anger comes out of being dependent on you. And you are healthy. But it doesn't register with them—the difficulty that *you* have in doing what you're doing.

Mr. Davis's use of the present and past tense in this account suggested that he relived the bitterness of these experiences. When asked if he was able to talk with anyone, such as his son, his in-laws, or clergy persons about the mounting pressures, he disclosed several reasons why he could not.

> My son came occasionally (to visit), but he worked and he had children. He did the best he could because some people can't handle illness of a loved one. And I wouldn't speak to my in-laws because she (wife) had poisoned them against me. All this was constant. Then you have the pressure from having to put the medicine in her heart. It was unbelievable. No, I don't recall complaining to anyone about anything. I guess that's because it's my nature not to burden anyone with what I'm going through. Because I survived all the years on my own.

Mr. Davis brought up a central issue in caregiving. Past mutual affection between caregiver and care recipient proved key in caregivers experiencing a lessened sense of burden and a greater sense of satisfaction in caregiving (Black, 2010; Brummet & Dilworth-Anderson, 2012). The men we interviewed offered variations of this statement—"She'd be taking care of me if it was the other way around"—to show that the foundation of their caregiving was reciprocal love and concern. Mr. Davis's circumstances diverged from this model. Mrs. Davis's succession of illnesses had, Mr. Davis reported, "changed her personality." He felt estranged from his in-laws and was reluctant to involve his son in his own distress. Additionally, a significant aspect of Mr. Davis's isolation in caregiving was the identity he constructed as a youngster. He perceived himself as someone who "survives on his own and does not burden others" with problems.

When asked what the best thing was about being a caregiver, Mr. Davis replied:

> The best thing about being a caregiver for me was doing things [caregiving duties] without being criticized. You know the lack of appreciation was always there. You saw no appreciation in the face, in the tone of voice; you didn't see it in a word of encouragement or anything.

Mr. Davis depicted his wife, due to several long-term illnesses, as resentful of his good health and work success, marking their relationship as adversarial. He also distanced himself from her by saying "the face" or "the voice" when talking about her words or facial expressions. When asked if he had thought of himself as a caregiver, Mr. Davis responded:

> I don't think so, maybe years later, but we never thought of ourselves like that. We always took care of our own. Even as a kid, my mother was always taking care of somebody else. Somebody was always in our home that needed help. There was no nursing home in the African-American community, no such things as facilities for taking care of people. In the South it was just natural for us to take care of someone else.

In his response, Mr. Davis reached back and assumed the cultural identity of his ancestors. He then added, "So, we just thought of being responsible for the person in your life. You are married and 'for better or for worse, for richer or poorer, til death do us part.'"

Similar to Mr. Brunson, Mr. Davis recalled that the marriage vow, "til death do us part," drove the inevitability of caring for one's spouse. Yet the same words infer different emotions to the listener. Duty and love are implied in both men's commitment, but perhaps in different measure.

AGING, IDENTITY, AND CAREGIVING

The characteristics of identity and caregiving in a primary caregiver come together in a singular way in older age. As seen in this chapter, for some persons, a personal identity became crystallized early in life (Horowitz, 2012). Families of origin bequeathed beliefs or principles that shaped men's patterns of behavior in childhood and acted as lenses through which family and community illness and need were viewed. Yet identity is constructed complexly. External changes in men's lives, based on new or altered contexts, such as a wife's or mother's illness, led to men's reassessments of roles and a reconstruction of identity, which showed a continuing process of development in older age (Hopp & Thomas, 2014). Although the bulwark of men's self-definitions resonated with a masculine standard, masculinities were not "fixed" in the men interviewed. The arduous, humbling, and overwhelming tasks of caregiving made a loose fit of traditional masculine behaviors when respondents were faced with ill wives or mothers who needed their care (Hanlon, 2012).

There are no stereotypical caregivers. Men seemed to continually reevaluate their self-perception based on new evidence about oneself, others, and the amount and type of work involved in caregiving. The context that bracketed caregiving, that is, men's smaller world of home and family, was especially fluid, shaped by the nature and progression of the care recipient's illness and the resultant changes in her abilities and personality (Hasselkus & Murray, 2007; Lane & King, 2012). Also, "when" in life the care recipient became debilitated, how long the caregiver had been giving care, and other circumstances that competed for attention during this time, such as working outside the home or giving care to another person, were significant in men's discussion of if and how they perceived themselves as caregivers. The most important disclosures of men's caregiving identities were their self-appraisals as caregivers, the descriptions of the care they gave, and why they did so (Pierre et al., 2001).

Mr. Gilmore and Mr. Brunson invested the moral principles they learned in childhood into their responsibilities throughout life and applied them to caregiving. For both men, particular values were revealed through continuing themes in their narratives, such as Mr. Gilmore's strong work ethic and Mr. Brunson's adherence to "keeping his word" in all situations. For both men, present-day patterns of behavior in caregiving rested on inherited traditions.

Mr. Gilmore "worked hard" in caregiving. He combined the care he saw given to elders in his home with devotion to Donna, his sensitivity to how he appeared as a caregiver to the wider world, and to his ability to morally imagine the emotional and physical suffering of aphasia. He acknowledged the importance of personal memory and the pain he and Donna felt in *her* being unable to voice those memories.

Both Mr. Brunson and Mr. Parker applied their long-established moral code of honesty to marriage and caregiving. Although neither Mr. Brunson nor Mr. Parker witnessed caregiving in their homes as youngsters, they performed the tasks of caregiving as a way of honoring their marriage vows and affirming that they were accomplishing "what needed to be done." Mr. Brunson acquired a strong sense of "we" in his family of origin and thrived as a caregiver through feelings of "belonging" with others—his wives, children, coworkers, and neighbors.

Although Mr. Kelch had not participated in caregiving as a youngster and assumed it was "woman's work," he amended his opinion to meet a personal necessity in life—giving care to his wife. He knew the type of father he wanted to be to his children, and the husband he must be for his wife. He therefore revised the role of father to include being an advocate for his children, and he added intensive physical care to his definition of marital love when his wife became ill.

Mr. Stokes kept, in the latter part of his life, the traditions that he inherited from his mother and honored them by giving her care. He mentioned throughout the interview that he viewed caregiving as an "education" that expanded his view of himself. He realized, he said, that it is "not until you change your whole routine" for someone that your words about caregiving "are not empty."

Research shows that a critical component in a caregiver's satisfaction is his conviction that the care recipient appreciates him (Snellman et al., 2012). Four of the men discussed in this chapter found satisfaction in caregiving despite the difficulty of particular tasks. Although this was not the case for Mr. Davis, his narrative strongly resonated with the African-American moral stance of caring for one's own. We note that, while giving care to his wife, Mr. Davis worked at two jobs to pay for his wife's medical bills. He also had little to no support from others. Mr. Davis took on, however, an African-American group identity. For many people, the legacy of family acts as a frame within which a personal identity takes form. Because of the illness of his mother and the emotional distance of his father, Mr. Davis had neither the backdrop of family tradition nor kin who could offer support. He gleaned a personal identity from the finest group characteristics he perceived in African-American culture and from African-American heroes he emulated (Thomas, 2012).

Giving daily personal care to a loved one can change mundane or unpleasant chores into a role that integrates identity (Black et al., 2008; Micka, 2006; Thomas, 2012). For the men discussed here, caregiving transformed their multiple tasks into an internal process of morally imagining the suffering of the care recipient. The comingling of aging, identity, and caregiving is complex. A caregiver's experience of the moral rightness of giving care to a loved one provided, in part, meaning for the most difficult of caregiving tasks. This sense of doing what was "right" was a symbolic theme that retrospectively threaded all roles and stages of the caregiver's life (Luborsky, 1993), and affirmed him as a good husband, son, worker, and caregiver.

In the next chapter we explore the phenomenon of generativity in our caregiving men. We suggest that men's identity and their attitudes and behaviors of generativity are linked particularly through giving care to another. It is also through the personal and communal identity discussed in this chapter that men revealed the unique modes and outlets of their generativity.

CHAPTER 3

Caregiving and Generativity

The concept of generativity evolved in the years following the presentation of Erikson's (1963) definition of generativity as "mature individuals' interest in guiding the next generation." Decades later, Erikson readdressed the life cycle concept in his older age, expanded the concept of generativity to include one's desire to care for others, to feel challenged, to be creative, and to be needed (Erikson, Erikson, & Kivnik, 1986). Later studies disclosed that generativity, as an individual's faith and hope for a world that will continue after personal death, has a broad scope, a long trajectory, and myriad outlets (Black, Hannum, Rubinstein, & DeMedeiros, 2015; Kotre, 2005; McAdams, 2012; Rubinstein, 1992; Rubinstein, Girling, de Medeiros, Brazda, & Hannum, 2014).

Research conducted early in the 21st century further expanded the definition of generativity and showed its contextualized nature. That is, each cohort's sense of generativity was shaped by the time and place into which its members were born. As mentioned throughout this book, the history of courageous distant ancestors, the guidance of parents and grandparents, and the present need of loved ones were implicated in African-American men's narratives of caregiving (Frazier, 1974). Caregivers talked about the long road from slavery to the civil rights marches of their younger days, and eventually to witnessing the election of the first African-American president in their later years. A picture of President Obama held a prominent place in many of our caregivers' homes.

Research has shown that generative interest in social causes usually develops early in life (Black et al., 2015). In relation to family legacy, the morality of caregiving is sown in childhood due to witnessing caregiving in the home (Black, 2010). Thus, our respondents' generative actions undergirded cultural, legal, political, and social issues (Aldwin & Gilmer, 2013; Gelder, 2007), and created outlets of concern about issues of justice, religion, art, and science (Baldwin, 1961; Black et al., 2015; Eisenhandler, 2003).

The heterogeneity of cultural groups, such as African Americans, makes broad statements about cultural generativity seem simplistic. Yet a group's cultural framework incorporates the sum of its experiences as a group, including those of the long past, into its current norms and values (Koltko-Rivera, 2004). In attempting to expand the definition of generativity based on the range of African-American older adults' lifestyles and changing contexts, our research investigated men's caregiving as a unique form of cultural and individual generativity.

The act of giving physical and emotional care to another is itself generative. In our group of African-American respondents, age, ethnicity, and gender influenced their caregiving attitudes and behaviors, which were culled from a lifetime of witnessing the moral and social value of giving kin or nonkin compassionate care. The nature and progression of care recipients' illness and debility determined men's specific areas of concern within caregiving. In our previous chapter, Mr. Gilmore's desire to physically care for his wife was nurtured early in life; it was fostered by the models of old age, debility, and need he witnessed within family and community. His wife's illness generated the actual care work he provided. Although generative attitudes and behaviors may be initiated as a family legacy, caregiving acts were shaped by the unique circumstances men encountered. The tasks each man accomplished, the scope of his responsibility, and the care recipient's level of impairment prompted creativity in the caregiving role. Each caregiver crafted a unique scenario of caregiving based on the context of his personal situation.

MR. CLAUDE GROSS

We introduce Mr. Claude Gross, aged 79, who lived with his wife of 59 years, Selina, in their large, multilevel North Philadelphia home. The couple had a daughter and son, both of whom lived nearby. Mr. Gross stood well over six and a half feet tall, was solidly built, and had dark hair. His size, his expansive personality, and his background as a semiprofessional basketball player who played with the Eastern League and traveled in diverse circles made him an engaging conversationalist. He retired from several careers he held throughout his life, such as a drug and alcohol counselor, an assistant with the Philadelphia school system, and an employee in the

US post office, but continued to coach youth basketball. He has coached in the Baker League, the Sonny Hill League, the Future League, and the Development League. He also coached a girls' basketball team. Although his work with youth highlights him as a principal character for research on generativity, it was for his role as his mother's caregiver that we include him in this chapter.

Mr. Gross was the primary caregiver for his mother who suffered from the effects of Alzheimer's disease. As mentioned in our first chapter, the circumstance of an elder child caring for a parent will become increasingly prevalent as the population ages. Older adults who themselves are facing acute or chronic health issues will be providing physical and emotional care for very old relatives. Mr. Gross's situation shows that definitions of generativity, once considered actions and expressions toward offspring and the young, were expanded to include nurturance toward the older generation. When asked how long he had cared for his mother, Mr. Gross replied:

> Ah, I would say longer than 4 years, but during that time I got to confusing dementia and Alzheimer's. Before that I could see some differences in her, but you give care to make things all right. I shop for her, talk with her. Me and her was really tight, and so for maybe 5 years she was in the Alzheimer's thing. But it took a while for me to pick that up, what was happening.

Although Mr. Gross witnessed a cognitive decline in his mother, his initial "caregiving" began as a way to maintain the status quo, that is, to help his mother preserve her independence by remaining in her own home. For Mr. Gross, it was difficult to discern exactly when her lapses in memory or judgment indicated a more serious condition. Asked when he realized "what was happening," Mr. Gross replied:

> I live around the corner from her (mother's home). She's in a 14-room house, right? And there were people knocking on her door and asking for cigarettes and stuff. I gave her—her sign is Gemini—a gold medallion [to wear] and it wasn't around her neck. "What happened to it?" She couldn't tell me. Ah, people were coming in [her house]. She said, "Oh, they so nice." They'd be borrowing two, three dollars from her. The crack people were coming. Then I take charge. My brother lives around the corner but nobody ah . . . One mother can take care of 13 children but 13 children can't take care of one mom. Ah, they (siblings) are working and they can't get there till 6 o'clock and ah, no transportation. Me and my wife and daughter was on call for my mother.

Mr. Gross hired an aide experienced with dementia patients, but his mother was eligible for this assistance only 4 hours a day. He strategized in order to keep her "covered" the rest of the time.

> I had to figure out what I can do after 4 hours. Get her (mother) washed in the morning, and fed. She liked to sit in the living room chair. I said to the lady (aide), "If you leave at noon and it take an hour to travel someplace else, that hour I'd like to keep, so I'll drive you." It worked out. She gave me all the extra time she had. She ate there so she didn't need no lunch.

Mr. Gross described this aide as his "partner" in caring for his mother.

> I helped her with salary. I gave her money and transportation because she took care of my mother, and that was precious for me. I would go get her if necessary; I would do anything to make it worth her while. I felt assured that my mother was getting care when I wasn't there. I didn't look to my brothers and sisters [to help with my mother's care]. I just worked with this lady.

Mr. Gross believed that their history together made them especially "tight." When asked how he came to be her primary caregiver, he responded:

> Me and my mom—I think I'm going to be a little selfish—was tighter than my brothers and sisters. We went through a lot of stuff. You realize that I was the baby for 12 years, which means I am with her more before the second branch of children were born (Mr. Gross is the youngest of his parent's first four children; 12 years separate him from the birth of his next sibling). I am around her more. I went to her job. She ironed shirts for this Chinese laundry; I worked in the Chinese restaurant which all my family worked for the same two cousins.

With the aide's help, Mr. Gross monitored his mother's cognitive and physical health. When asked if her personality "changed," with dementia, Mr. Gross laughed. He recalled how she disregarded doctors' questions that she deemed irrelevant:

> I'll tell you a story. I took her to all these doctors to find out where she was (cognitively and physically). I took her to the dentist, the eye doctor, the psychiatrist. The psychiatrist asked her, "Do you know the current president?" She said, "What's that got to do with anything?" And socked the shit out of him (laughter). The psychiatrist said, "You ain't gonna let nobody fool you." But she started getting angry more. She only didn't get angry when she was comfortable

around certain people. That's a human thing. Here's an analogy. A dog hears a certain voice or scent, they relax. You hear him say, "Grrrr," that mean he can't figure it out, so he get angry. Now, she didn't know the doctor, but she loved the lady (aide). Was it in her mind this lady was helping her? I don't know. She'd always say to me, "Is everything all right, Claude?" I said, "Sure, Mom, we got the right people here."

He thoughtfully tracked his mother's cognitive awareness, pondered its meaning, and used real-world analogies for interpreting it to himself and others. The most profound outlet of Mr. Gross's generativity was his enduring attention to his mother's welfare. It began in a childhood that included spending time at her workplace, and it lasted well into Mr. Gross's older age. We will revisit Mr. Gross in a later chapter.

MR. LOUIS COLBERT

Mr. Louis Colbert, aged 62, was interviewed in his home. As a senior administrator and social worker for an older adult agency, he is dedicated particularly to the well-being of low-income elders. In his day-to-day job he works closely with those who care for elders, such as care managers, nurses, and formal and informal caregivers. It is, however, for his work (with his siblings) as a caregiver, that we include him in this chapter.

Mr. Colbert, along with six siblings, gave care to their mother in the family home until her passing. When asked to describe his mother, he smiled.

My mom was about 5'6" and always on a diet. She wasn't obese; she was healthy. She was optimistic, she had a beautiful smile, and there was no such thing as a hidden agenda with her. What you saw is what you got. But if you messed with her kids, a whole side of her—that I seldom saw—would come out and she could kick your ass. And I never, ever, ever, ever remember hearing my mother say she did not like somebody.

In a few descriptive sentences, Mr. Colbert offered a vivid picture of a vital woman. Mr. Colbert said she had endured several illnesses throughout her older age, including diabetes, high blood pressure, and Parkinson's disease. Toward the end of her life, she also suffered from dementia. He traced the beginning of his mother's decline to the demise of his father.

The last summer my father was alive he kept saying, "Something don't feel right. I need to go to the doctor. But I got to get these projects done for your

> mother. Once I finish, then I'll go. Finally in November he goes to the doctor and he (doctor) basically says to him, "You've got pancreatic cancer." So that's November; February he was dead. And I remember the day after he died my mother came downstairs; she was in the living room and her hand was shaking real bad. I never seen it shake like that. So (pause) she had about (pause) 2 good years after that 'cause she was still driving. But that in my head was the beginning of the decline—my father's illness and death. So it's like the visible and the invisible thing. I think it's hard emotionally to be married to somebody for over 50 years and then that person is gone. I think it takes a while to get used to that space not being filled up, if you ever get used to it.

This poignant comment reveals Mr. Colbert's understanding of the holistic nature of health and illness. His mother's grief, along with her physical ills, precipitated a decline that surprised Mr. Colbert in its swiftness.

> It's just now that it seems to me that my mother went from being ambulatory and driving, then she decided to give up the keys. So she quit driving and she moved into the category of frail elderly—it seemed to me—rather fast.

When asked how he came to be his mother's primary caregiver, Mr. Colbert laughed. He noted that although all seven children cared for their mother, his personal characteristics pushed him to the fore.

> Well, I tend to have the biggest mouth. What happened was when my mother first got to where she was bedbound, the hospital bed was downstairs, and we had this informal care plan where the sisters were doing everything and the brothers stepped back and let them do it. Part of that involved my younger sister who worked from mom's house and take care of mom at the same time. That lasted for about a month because mom was disruptive (laughs). That just doesn't work! "I got to go to the bathroom. I got to pee. I want to eat." So my sister was reaching out and we were all kind of ignoring her 'til we got an e-mail one day: "This is not working. We have to put Mom in a nursing home."

Mr. Colbert assessed that the burden of a parent's care often falls on one child (usually a daughter). As a social worker, he knew that family members' good intentions to share the labor can fall short during the days, months, and years of caregiving. Although one of our caregivers said accurately, "It takes a team to care for my wife," it is usually not the case for a caregiver to have a team. It is not surprising that Mr. Colbert's sister soon realized their mother needed full-time care. What is uncommon is how the rest of the Colbert family responded.

> That got everybody's attention (laughs). At that point I kind of stepped up and said, "Okay, let me do what I do best." 'Cause I'm the middle of seven, and my Mom always said I was the bossiest of all her kids (laughs). I tend to be the mouthpiece. I brought everybody together and said, "It's as simple as this: We have to do a schedule, a chart." It started with my oldest brother, Bernard. We paid him to be there at 7:00 in the morning when my sister went to work. My oldest sister lived at the house. Bernard was there until the home health aide got there, about 9:00. She would bathe her, give her breakfast, get her dressed. On the days Mom went to Adult Day Care, the van picked her up at 10:00 in a van. My job was I'd be there at 4:30 waiting for that van to drop her off. On weekends we took turns. So basically she was never left alone.

Mr. Colbert said that the family met every 3 months to assess their timetable and discover "what was working; what wasn't." This intricate family schedule required family dedication and cooperation. Mr. Colbert said that his Mother had been a model for giving care to others.

> Next door to our house in Media was these three old ladies from West Chester. One of them died; there was two left and one of them was blind. My Mother would cook for the night and one of the kids would bring two plates over there. If they had to go to the doctor, my dad would take them, or when he cut our lawn, he'd cut their lawn. My Mom was a tremendous role model in terms of faith in God. It's about helping people in need.

Mr. Colbert remembered the ubiquity of old people in everyday life when he was growing up.

> Old people were always around us. Where we grew up in the country, it was very isolated. My Grandmother grew up in that house. She had two sisters and we were all close. Seven Black homes all together. All of those were like my Grandmother's cousins. When somebody needed help, you helped. What I think I understand now is that was the helping tradition that is so real in the African-American family [and] that is passed on from one generation to another.

As a professional, Mr. Colbert was familiar with the plethora of issues that surround old age and caregiving. Yet, when his Mother became ill, he acknowledged that "years and years of experience" could not have prepared him adequately for the acts involved in giving care to a beloved Mother, particularly those surrounding toileting and hygiene. Mr. Colbert mentioned that "even experts" on aging and caregiving, until they have cared for their own, are visitors in this strange land. In fact, Mr. Colbert did not think of himself as a caregiver. He explained.

> We are educated and we are smart. You know I run a caregivers' support group. I was two years into caregiving, two years into the process before it dawned on me that *I* was a caregiver. It never clicked in my head, never! It's different when it's a husband taking care of the wife, as compared to when it's Mother and son. It's very, very, very . . . (does not complete sentence). I will always remember the first time I had to take my Mother to the bathroom. My oldest brother, her first child, he could never do it.

Similar to many other respondents in this study, the most onerous feature of caregiving surrounded the issue of elimination and incontinence. When Mr. Colbert was asked about his favorite aspect of giving care to his other, he smiled:

> She came home from daycare at 4:30. I'm waiting. We have a ramp, she comes in. "Mom, go to the bathroom. Do you want something to eat." I didn't want her to go to bed, so, "Do you want to watch tv?" The dementia had gotten to the point where that was not registering. She wheeled herself into the kitchen and opened cabinets and pulled out pots. "Mom, what are you doing?" "I'm making apple pie." Then, after awhile, she'd want to lay down and I'd say, "Do you want to sit up?" "Yeah, I want to sit up." She would sit on the side of the bed and you just sit there next to her and just hold her. You know she was at that stage where she knew who you were, and then she moved to the stage where she knew you were a male relative, but didn't know if you were brother, son, husband, father (pause). But she knew she was safe. And then she would move to the realm where it was just, it was the spirit you could feel . . . like, she'd be sitting and you'd have your arm around her and she would just put her head on your shoulder and you could feel her being relaxed (pause). Yeah, because she knew she was safe. That was always the important thing—knowing she was in that space and she wasn't in pain.

Mr. Colbert exemplified generativity in his professional work with elders. It was his concern for his mother's comfort and safety that provided us with an inside look at a unique aspect of generativity: Although his mother was nearing the end stage of life, he knew that she continued to desire and deserve his time, touch, and presence.

Mr. Gross and Mr. Colbert addressed the primal fear of a care recipient when she no longer recognizes loved ones or feels threatened by the perceived strangeness of her surroundings. One of the last and most important gifts these caregivers gave to their mothers was helping them feel "safe." Each man's mother clearly communicated her personhood in feeling protected by her son's presence (Volicer & van der Steen, 2014).

MR. ALEXANDER EL

We introduce Mr. Alexander El, aged 68, who was interviewed in the West Philadelphia home he shared with his wife, Lois. Mr. El, who stood tall and slender, wore African dress in the Moorish-American tradition. His voice was deep and soft; he spoke slowly and gave careful thought to his answers. Mr. El was a jazz percussionist who at one point during the interview described playing and composing music as "like breathing." The couple's home was filled with colorful art that Mr. El painted. In an interesting aside, when the first author began to listen to the audio recording of Mr. El's interview, soft piano jazz, composed and performed by Mr. El, came through the recorder. It was reminiscent of stones skipping on water or skates gliding over ice.

Mr. El grew up in South Philadelphia with a coterie of talented musicians. The musicians welcomed the young people and encouraged them to listen to music and practice constantly. It was an dynamic locale for the groundbreaking jazz music that came out of Philadelphia in the 1950s and 1960s. Mr. El remembered being mentored in the neighborhood jam sessions by men who eventually became world-class musicians.

> We were a village and raised as a village. The neighborhood raised me. Hard-working people work, come home, and take care of your property. If there were anything negative in my upbringing, it was my doing (laughs). I was bull-headed, stubborn.

Mr. El, as a young teenager, along with his brother, gave care to their mother. When asked how he and his brother came to be their mother's caregivers, he replied, "My mother had what I call the other terrible disease, Parkinson's. She had medical help but basically it was me and my brother who took care of her." After a pause, Mr. El looked away from the interviewer, into the distance that was his early life.

> When I think back, I didn't really know what I was doing at the time. The odd thing about that is that we weren't used to needing health professionals. I mean parents, they got sick and then they got better and got up and did their work. I was a young man. I was involved in a lot of different things. First it was my father. He had fell, and he eventually died from the fall. The first thing I noticed

> with my mother was that once when she was cooking, I asked her why her hand was shaking. She said, "Oh, it's probably just tired."

Mr. El was saddened by the memories of his father's early demise and his mother's illness. Although he and his brother were her primary caregivers, they were little prepared for the role. He mentioned that, like all youngsters, "you think your parents will always be there." In retrospect, the brothers could not know how the disease would progress and what they would face as it worsened.

Mr. El: It was a sad situation. And it was a hard time for the family. My one brother was married and my sister had problems with her health. I always felt if I knew more about the disease, I could have done more. But it wasn't like today, with the miracle of the computer. My only regret is that if I had known about the disease . . .

Interviewer: How did you come to be her caregiver?

Mr. El: I would say the motivating issue was that it needed to be done . . . but I call it an honor to take care of her. It's like when you put on your shoes. My mom was the shoe. I was the laces; I had to tie her up (pause). But I wish I could have done better, even now. Even today, I could be taking care of her.

This interesting metaphor of the shoe and the laces inferred to the listener that the shoe and the laces complete each other, with the shoe being the foundational item. Yet the laces become more necessary to hold the shoe together as the shoe grows old, wears out, and begins to come apart.

Throughout his life, Mr. El's great passion was music. Having sat at the feet of jazz greats and honing his talent since youth, Mr. El eventually worked as a jazz musician. After his mother's death, he described how he met his wife.

> I was working as a musician in Lansdowne. At that time people of color were starting to go skiing and there was a dance to take place after skiing. Well, there was a snowstorm, so nobody came, not the rest of the band either. I was the only one. But she (Lois) was there. So there was a lot of people trying to figure out why we didn't meet before this because we were in the same social circle.

The couple brought Lois's mother into their home after she was diagnosed with Alzheimer's disease. In contrast to his perceived lack of skill in caring for his own mother as a youth, Mr. El spoke with pride about giving care to his mother-in-law, whom he called "Mom."

Mr. El: Her name was Madeline. She was a teacher, a nurse, opera singer, church activist, always on the go, which is similar to my wife (laughter). A beautiful, warm, vibrant person. She came to live with us because of her illness. Basically we had taken her out of her house because she was unable to take care of it. Now this was similar to Parkinson's in its effects. But Parkinson's is more a physical attack on the brain. Alzheimer's starts with deterioration of the brain and affects the mind.

Interviewer: Was there a difference in giving care to your mother and your mother-in-law?

Mr. El: Yes, I was more there for my mother-in-law. I was older, and age does make a difference.

Although painful to recall, Mr. El's recollection that he had probably fallen short in caring for his mother supplied the impetus to give loving care to his mother-in-law. Although the illness and death of his mother may have helped form his identity as a caregiver, the picture he painted of himself at the time of his mother's illness is blurry. Perhaps caring for Lois's mother was akin to a second chance to care for a loved one with a devastating illness, but this time he was equal to the task. The care that he and his wife gave Lois's mother seemed to reflect his competence in caregiving and his maturity as a man.

An individual's generativity, or what he offers to others from his storehouse of knowledge or skills, is also revealed by the goals he keeps or creates in the sixth or seventh decade of life. We return to Mr. Gilmore. He reported that he was aware that persons of all colors and ethnicities "watched" how he cared for his aphasic wife. He approached caregiving—and life itself—as a representative of African-American men. For Mr. Gilmore, giving care to his wife showed the larger world who he was as an individual and as a member of a group. His present goal revealed the wide range of his generativity.

> I look at race relations around the world. I'm 60 years old and tired of the hatred. But I hate that people categorize me as an Afro-American. When they see on the news we are thugs and don't take care of our families—that make me go out every day and strive to be the best I can. I wonder why I have to do this, but this is my goal: I try to get along with all races. I've gone out of my way to speak

> to the White man and the Asians I know don't like us. I don't kiss your butt; if I see you're a bigot and don't want to associate with me, I move on. So my goal now is to have a better relationship with all races. This world is big enough for all. This isn't a one-man university; it's a university of all mankind. So even though I'm stereotyped—all Afro-American males aren't what you see on the news every day.

Mr. Gilmore felt an internal push to show African-American men as diverse in knowledge, varied in skills, and driven by concerns about family, community, and the world—and not as one-dimensional figures viewed on news reports. In past research, African-American elder males acted as representatives for their cohort for at least two reasons: (1) pride in self, gratitude for an African-American legacy that included family and community strength, and a desire to promote pride and gratitude in other men and (2) as a living example of Du Bois's "double consciousness." Mr. Gilmore's agreement to be interviewed for this book sprang, in part, from a desire to transform long-held negative stereotypes about African-American men. He offered a window into his life as a husband and caregiver, and shared his goals as an African-American man.

Our caregiving men recognized that oppression and deprivation in our country and world was immeasurable. Yet, they focused their generative behavior most intently on where they could serve the best—in their own homes and neighborhoods.

MR. CHARLIE WAYNS

We present Mr. Charlie Wayns, a 76-year-old retiree, as an exemplar of generativity in his community. Mr. Wayns was a tall, slender man with deep brown skin who wore glasses. On the day of the interview he sported a baseball cap. Mr. Wayns had taken on the responsibility of caring for several people, including his wife of 53 years, Joan, and Joan's mother, who lived nearby, along with several neighbors in his Philadelphia neighborhood.

In walking through Mr. Wayns's home, which he renovated and remodeled, the interviewer noted that the dining room table was formally set. Mr. Wayns explained that, although no guests were expected, "It's been a tradition since we came up as children. The table was always set, ready for company to have a meal." When asked if he and his wife eat dinner at the dining table, he laughed, "Ninety percent of the time we eat in the kitchen." The presentation of his home and its traditions showed the impact of his parents' legacy and his intent to bequeath that legacy to his children.

When asked, Mr. Wayns talked about the care his wife required.

> She had a hip replacement and it's a matter of time 'til she gets the knee replaced. She's getting slower every day and I'm always around when she needs me. Plus I take care of my mother-in-law, who's 93. We spend a lot of time taking her to doctors and seeing she gets what she needs. I have a sister, she got frostbitten years ago and had both legs amputated. She's been in the nursing home for a long time, and we go see her constantly. We take her out when we can.

A neighbor described Mr. Wayns to the interviewer as "a male Florence Nightingale. Whenever people run into problems, he's there to assist. He's a part-time caregiver for a whole lot of people." When the interviewer repeated this description, Mr. Wayns smiled.

> I like to help out in the neighborhood, but I don't take on no long jibbity things cause between her (wife's) and her mother, they come first. But I try to help senior citizens. Larry Wilson is my good friend; he's a wonderful neighbor. I do anything I can for him. There's a lady around the street; Miss Jackson is 93. She lives by herself and I take her to the doctor, pick up medicine, do things in the house for her. I put her hot water heater in; I fixed her toilet and her sink. She's so appreciative. We all need help, but when you're old and don't have nowhere to turn, it's a big problem.

Men's generativity, like Mr. Wayns's, occurred in the natural settings of their lives—home, neighborhood, and work. The people who dwelled in these small spaces were the foci of generative attitudes and behaviors. They invested the talents they possessed or skills learned earlier in life to ease the hardship of family, friends, and neighbors. We have elsewhere named persons' every day, practical acts of compassion for those who are ill, infirm, or elderly "the power of the little" (Black et al., 2008). Although the next generation has been considered the major repository for generative actions and behaviors, personal ingenuity, empathy, and generativity are disclosed through the homegrown ways our respondents gave care to those who are their own age and older.

MR. LARRY WILSON

We next introduce the neighbor that Mr. Wayns mentioned, Mr. Larry Wilson. Mr. Wilson was a 78-year-old widower who cared for his wife,

Mercedes, until her death. Mr. Wilson was outside when the interviewer climbed his front steps and greeted him. Mr. Wilson said hello and, in what seemed like an unconscious act, picked up a watering can and sprinkled the flowers in the front garden. This small gesture seemed symbolic, representative of the manner in which Mr. Wilson cultivated all areas of his life. Now retired, he had worked as an Industrial Coordinator for a local university. Along with this full-time job, Mr. Wilson also coached a track team on Saturdays and played the drums in his brother's band on weekend evenings.

> I stopped playing in the band in '83. We played every Friday night—I'd get home at 3:00 in the morning and get up around 7:00 to meet the track team I was coaching, and stayed at the track meet all day. I'd come home, get dressed Saturday night to go play in the band. I did it for about 20 years. In fact, what happened was we were at a job, on stage with a curtain backdrop playing this up-tempo jazz song, and I fell asleep and fell off the stage. I disappeared behind the curtain. My brother said, "Larry, you need to make a decision. Do you want to coach or play?" But he knew coaching was my heart. So I said, "I'm going to give up playing in the band."

Mr. Wilson continued to coach the girls' track team at Gwynedd Mercy Academy. "I coach track and cross country. We're getting ready for a track meet tomorrow. I think we should win it," he added proudly. When asked about his current health, he smiled.

> You know, I'm getting old, and you start to slow down. I am just blessed to get out of bed, do my chores. I'm painting now, and today I was planting flowers which I like. I try to keep my house up. My parents kept a neat house; my wife kept a neat house. The things that are around here, the great memories of her [wife], (points to sofa cushions) like these, she had them made.

When asked to describe his wife, he replied:

> I admired her. I married a woman who had four kids. So I have four kids, eight grandkids, and three great grandkids. My wife had them before we got married. So they are my stepkids, but I consider them my kids.

Mr. Wilson was the primary caregiver for his wife Mercedes for over 14 years. She was diagnosed with Alzheimer's disease in the late 1990s; he retired 2 years later to be her full-time caregiver. He recalled his first inkling that something was wrong.

> I didn't know much about Alzheimer's when I found out that's what she had. The way I found out, one day I was mopping the floor underneath the sofa in the living room and her shoes were under there. I said, that's strange that she hid them. Another day I was in my closet. I looked behind my sweaters and her shoes were there. So we took her to the doctor and he diagnosed her with dementia. She had to retire because she did a lot of traveling for her job and she got lost once. So things just started getting worse.

Mercedes's behavior was not unusual in care recipients who are in the earlier stages of dementia. Hiding personal items, or believing missing items had been stolen by neighbors or visitors to the home, signaled a problem that usually "get deeper" with time. When asked how he came to be Mercedes's primary caregiver, Mr. Wilson reported that he discussed her care with the children.

> I sat my daughters and son down; we were sitting right at this table and I told them, "Your mother has Alzheimer's. It will probably deteriorate as time goes by. But I don't want her to go to a nursing home. I'm going to take care of her." It was my choice to be the primary caregiver. I was her husband. I wanted to make sure she was taken care of by me. I didn't want her to go to any nursing home (begins to cry).

Mercedes stayed in their home until her passing. After her death he asked his brother to move in with him. "I said, 'Wayne, I got space here. Why don't you come on and live here?' I'm glad he did cause it's company for me."

Similar to Mr. Wayns and the traditions he continued in his home, such as keeping the dining table set, Mr. Wilson also mentioned a tradition Mercedes enjoyed, and that he continued.

> I set up the Christmas decorations in memory of my wife. Her birthday was on the 28th of November, so I would start early and turn the lights on that night. She always liked the way I decorated the house so I do it every year. It's getting more difficult, although Wayne helps me quite a bit. I don't go up in the trees like I used to. I just try to keep my kids coming. I say to them, "Come over tonight 'cause it's your mother's birthday and I'm turning the Christmas lights on in her memory."

The interviewer noted that Mr. Wilson's decorated house at Christmastime is anticipated by the entire neighborhood. It is reminiscent of the lights and animation of former Philadelphia department store windows like Gimbel Brothers, Lit Brothers, and Snellenbergs.

Mr. Wilson channeled the faithful care of his wife into their home, which became a repository of his memories and a symbol of their "good life" together. He attends to those features—flowers in the garden and Christmas decorations—that represent her ongoing presence in his life. When asked about current goals, Mr. Wilson answered:

> I want to stay here in my home. My goal is to try to stay as healthy as possible, to support the kids and to keep the closeness I have with my sisters and brothers. My parents would be very proud.

Mr. Wilson seemed to stand in the center of a continuum of care and nurturance that stretched back to his parents and grandparents and forward to his children and grandchildren. His generativity was shown by his devotion to his wife, her children, and his brothers and sisters. It is currently manifested by attention to his home, which seemed to keep Mercedes close by. We will revisit Mr. Wilson in a later chapter.

THE MANY FACES AND FACETS OF GENERATIVITY

Men's early experiences, especially those that occurred in multigenerational households, led to memories of giving care to elders as "just the normal thing" or "just the way it was." Culturally generative attitudes and behaviors were internalized through childhood lessons of keeping the aged and infirm close within the family circle. Discussion of how, when, where, and why men gave care to beloved others revealed the internal processes of men's decisions to take on caregiving. For most men, caregiving, even if they did not label it such, was "nothing out of the ordinary."

Mr. Gross explained that his mother maintained her ability to sense comfort or danger while in the throes of dementia. He thus revealed an important fortification against "the lost self" (Ribeiro et al., 2007) syndrome of mental disease or defect. Mr. Gross's believed that despite cognitive impairment, his mother remained "herself" and primordially aware of safety or risk. In spite of her memory loss, Mr. Gross infused his mother, particularly in the stories he told about her, with the identity he long held of her (Kitwood, 1997).

Mr. Colbert, similar to Mr. Gross, considered that helping his mother "feel safe" despite advanced dementia was significant in his caregiving. He also did not identify his mother's inability to recognize him as indicative of loss of her personhood. Even after she began to "stare at the ceiling," he described her spirit as coming to the forefront of her self.

Mr. El experienced a particular type of generativity in his youth. The musicians in his neighborhood welcomed him to watch and learn their art. He also endured confusion and stress during his initial period of caregiving when he and his brother, at young ages, were responsible for the care of their mother, who had Parkinson's disease. Although the family had "professional help," he recalled how the medical and social sciences failed to develop a holistic care of persons with this illness. His ability and desire to care for his mother-in-law later in his life became for him a kind of redemption, although he did not use that word. He extended to her the grace and sensitivity that he most certainly would have given his mother.

Mr. Gilmore expanded notions of generativity to include promoting dialogues about race with "Whites and Asians." His portrait of himself as a hard worker, devoted husband, and caregiver revealed his belief in the "power of the little." If the entire community of African-American men can be judged by the deeds of one wrongdoer, he believed that the community also can be judged by his (and other men's) acts of inclusion.

Mr. Wayns also broadened the definition of generativity to include those who are not related to him and those who are older than he. Along with his wife, mother-in-law, and sister, Mr. Wayns felt responsibility toward older neighbors who needed assistance with everyday chores. He empathized with those who are ill, frail, alone, or unable to do what he, with gratitude, continued to accomplish—"just getting around."

Research on our respondents' generativity was constructed on the foundation of past research about generativity. In essence, we placed the construct of generativity within an existing framework (mentioned at the beginning of this chapter). Kotre (1985) extended previous definitions of generativity by identifying objects of generative action. That is, some persons invest themselves in a cherished project, object, or "thing" that they believe represents them, will outlive them, and can be passed on to others. This "object" may be inwardly and privately appreciated or shared with others. Mr. Wilson offered us a glimpse of this type of generative outlet. His home was an enduring expression of his love for Mercedes. Mr. El accomplished a similar manifestation of generativity with his music and art.

In our sample, generativity was often defined in terms of personal responsibility that had broad parameters. There were no age restrictions in regard to those who benefitted from our respondents' generativity, or persons or objects that fell outside of men's generative impulse. This impulse often began early in life and lasted into men's older age. Although caregiving was the primary way in which we studied men's generativity in this book, it was not the only way that men sought to invest themselves, and have faith in life and the world in which they lived.

Another way cultural generativity was conveyed within the community was for men to tell us about their lives, their work, and their caregiving. The men we interviewed offered narratives of caregiving that also were family stories about generativity. They showed the truth of the maxim that "no matter his or her span of influence, each individual can improve the world" (Black et al., 2011:42).

Our next chapter examines men's definitions and experiences of suffering. Each man revealed, in his interview, both the uniqueness and communality of suffering in the African-American community.

CHAPTER 4

Experiences of Suffering

Many persons, when interviewed for a prior study on the subject of suffering and asked to define or describe the word, spoke of physical pain. Intense bodily pain, or pain of long duration or uncertain origin, usually trumped thought and action regarding anything other than the pain. Some individuals spoke of suffering as the sense of anguish and hopelessness that accompanies depression or other mental illness. Yet, as each person recalled a physical injury, illness, or event as "painful," he also remembered feeling distress as a whole person—in body, mind, and spirit. With further probing, respondents' experiences of pain also included personal characteristics—that is, their ethnicity, personal biography, history, and current state of mental and physical health were integral to the experience and expression of pain. The context of pain—in what time of life it occurred, its cause, and its resolution or end—was also taken into account in whether the pain was defined as suffering.

As an example, an elderly African-American man named Mr. Darren was interviewed in the study mentioned earlier. He had been recently widowed. His responses to interview questions centered on feelings of loneliness after his wife's passing. Yet, when asked if there was an event, incident, or time period in life when he had suffered, he replied:

Mr. Darren: I really suffered with pain from ulcers. Mentally and physically. It was in the 70s. I was working at the arsenal. I had a fine engineering background and I don't get the promotion that Caucasians with the same background received. I couldn't achieve a breakthrough. That really got to me.

Interviewer: How did you come through that?

Mr. Darren: I had surgery for the ulcers. And I got an advancement, so that was a balm. I instituted an Equal Opportunity suit and took it all the way to Washington. They said I had to be placed in the position commensurate with my qualifications. And that was that.

Another African-American man, Mr. Wickers, interviewed for the same study, connected suffering with the pain of cancer that his wife experienced before she passed. With further probing, he said that illness, job loss, and a lack of compassion from his employers and the mortgage company that held the loan on his home contributed to his suffering.

> We bought a house. One of the kids got sick and I lost my job. I got behind in payments. I went to the mortgage people, see if I could pay interest 'til I catch up. They refused; I lost my home. We got an apartment, then she got cancer. Then I was on my own.

He perceived that underemployment, illness, and death robbed him of the strength to "keep fighting." He turned to history to relate the suffering inflicted on those who are considered "less than."

> The only people here in the beginning were Indians. No one can say the Indians were lined up on the east coast saying, "Come on over." And slavery, people being brought over from Africa and brutalized. Somewhere down the line someone has to pay for that.

Both men began their definitions of suffering as pain that evolved into an experience that ruptured the "self." Individuals' experiences of suffering varied, but most persons perceived that suffering included a sense, *due to external circumstances*, that they had been treated as less than a full human being. For Mr. Darren, suffering's resolution came from redress. For Mr. Wickers, no resolution occurred and the memory of this period haunted him decades later (Black, 2006).

For many African-American men born in the first half of the 20th century, the second reason for suffering mentioned earlier—a sense of feeling powerless—was an aspect of their everyday cultural and social history.

The internal battles waged in the mirrors of double consciousness posed threats to a man's loss of central life values, such as health or economic security, undermined self-integrity, and often led to a particular type of suffering related to feeling pulled apart, or living as if he were two persons.

One person, which was revealed to family and peers, was authentic and needed no explanation. The other was a persona constructed by the dominant culture.

Another African-American man interviewed for the study on suffering gave his interpretation of the word "suffering" for African-American men.

> At the beginning [of the "suffering" interview] I had a problem with the word "suffering" because I had a narrow concept of suffering. I thought you had to have physical suffering. But the emotional piece is what we deal with all the time. And that opened up a new window for me. Now I see suffering is emotional and within. It's the daily suffering, the daily hurt. There is no experience that we go through that isn't touched by race.

We present the above to show that suffering assaults an individual in the fullness of his personhood. The wholeness of his self feels ruptured. Because the main focus in this chapter is to explore the concept of suffering in relation to African-American elder male caregivers, we wondered whether one man's comment, that there is "no experience that is *not* touched by race" would hold true for our caregiving men and, if so, how they would address it. We revisit this question throughout this chapter and at its end.

The labor of caregiving is intense and all-consuming. A care recipient's illness or impairment usually includes diminished cognitive or physical abilities, which can be viewed as a deterioration of the care recipient's "self." The daily tasks of caregiving cause most caregivers to experience another characteristic of suffering—uncertainty over what comes next. How will the disease progress? What new symptoms will appear? Will I have the strength to remain a caregiver? What will happen if I die before her? In the case of Alzheimer's disease and other dementias, caregivers often cannot anticipate the startling manifestations of the disease, such as cursing, screaming, calling out in the night, crying through fear, confusion, paranoia, and ultimately the blank stare of not recognizing loved ones. Displays of anguish or panic may render socializing or attending religious services untenable. Expressivity (or its lack) in dementia may signal the beginning of isolation and a kind of social death for both the caregiver and care recipient (Moore, 2010).

As the care recipient's health and awareness wane, the tasks involved in caregiving increase. Caregivers may experience suffering due to the inherent paradox in caregiving. Caregiving responsibilities may cause caregivers to feel a certain loss of control over the circumstances of caregiving and of life. Both caregiver and care recipient may become demoralized as impairment advances. The physical tasks of caregiving, such as lifting or moving the loved one, pose risks to the care recipient and compromise the caregiver's health. The isolation of home caregiving can be catastrophic to an elder caregiver's emotional health (Anderson & Turner, 2010). An accumulated weariness may strike the caregiver and emerge as physical illness or depression (Brummet & Dilworth-Anderson, 2012) due to the labor and tedium of caregiving, a lack of respite, and the knowledge that the care recipient's mental and physical health will not improve.

Most men interviewed for this book assumed the task of caregiving willingly and felt supported by someone close to them—adult children, siblings, friends, or neighbors. Very few felt unsupported. Some men had secondary caregivers; others paid health aides on whom they relied. Aides often provided hands-on care for bathing and toileting, especially in the cases of men caring for their mothers. A few men relied on family, friends, neighbors, or fellow church members to stay with their loved one when necessary. One of our caregivers remarked that although he was grateful for even an hour's respite, he felt reluctant to leave the care recipient "for too long" because it was difficult for him to request help from others. For many caregiving men, it was the realization of the overwhelming responsibility—for making medical decisions, accidental falls or mishaps, or acknowledging that in the progression of the disease they saw the imminence of death—that caused a suffering unique to the caregiver.

Some caregivers said that perceived suffering by the loved one caused their own suffering. We return to Mr. Brunson who was introduced in Chapter Two, and who had cared for two wives in their final illnesses. When discussing the subject of suffering, Mr. Brunson recalled the day his first wife, Mattie, died.

> And her last day—she wanted to go to the shore, so we asked her doctor and he said, "Yeah, if she's up to it." So me and my youngest daughter took her to Wildwood. It was a Monday morning, and once we got there I pushed her in the wheelchair. And then she got sick. On our way back she asked God to take her home 'cause I guess she was tired of suffering.

For Mattie, there was no relief from nausea, pain, and weakness in her final weeks. With a minimalist elegance, Mr. Brunson described the extreme fatigue that represented her suffering and her prayer for it to end.

> When we got home, I cleaned her up because she had an accident and while we were doing that my daughter said, "Daddy, call the doctor." She said that Mattie's body was cleaning itself out; it was preparing for death. I didn't know

> how to answer that. So I lifted her up and ran out; me and my daughter took her to the hospital. And she died that afternoon. It was a hard journey.

Mr. Brunson used the word "suffering" to describe the waning of Mattie's body, mind, and spirit during the last stage of her life. He also described his bewilderment at being unable to understand the process of bodily death. He used the word "journey" to portray their visit to Wildwood *and* the trajectory of Mattie's illness. The word "home" described the house he shared with Mattie as well as their belief that heaven would be her final residence. When asked about the worst part of this journey, he replied:

> She was weighing 148 pounds when she was healthy, and when she died she was 85 pounds. 'Cause she couldn't eat. So, I guess the worst part was seeing her fade away. And there is nothing you can do.

An aspect of Mr. Brunson's suffering included his powerlessness at watching Mattie diminish throughout her illness and particularly at its end. He knew that the final step of this journey must be traveled by Mattie alone.

We return to Mr. Kelch, who we first met in Chapter Two, and who cared for his wife, Beverly, during her final illness. When asked how Beverly dealt with him being her primary caregiver, he replied:

> Well, at first [she was] uncomfortable because caregivers do everything and they get down and dirty and she would say, "Jim, I hate for you to see me like this. I never wanted you to see me like this." I said, "Love takes in everything, Beverly, you know, the good and the bad."

As the boundaries of the body break down during advanced illness, important personal values in our society are challenged. Autonomy, dignity, and privacy are stripped away as someone else becomes responsible for toileting, bathing, and dressing the care recipient. Mr. and Mrs. Kelch revealed the depth and complexity of emotion for both caregiver and care recipient as he gave, and she accepted, this level of care.

When asked about his physical health, Mr. Kelch replied that it was "good." When asked about his emotional health, he acknowledged that he suffered from "depression, sadness, melancholy." He reported that he was surprised by the depth of his emotions during and after his wife's illness and death, as well as by the number of years that have passed since she died.

> Seventeen years. It doesn't seem that long. I don't know how I've lasted without her, but ah, that's a big part of my, my ah, depression or whatever you

> want to call it. I, ah, I never thought I would outlive her, first of all. I prepared everything—made sure she would be well taken care of. Now it's come down to me being without her. I sometimes don't know how to live. But ah, you know you must go on. The kids and I talk about this frequently. We all share the pain. But I live in the hope I will see her again.

Mr. Kelch, like several of our respondents, believed that his wife would outlive him. He therefore described caregiving as a two-pronged period of his life. "I feel that I honored my wife by caring for her. But I know her life was not pleasurable towards the end. But making it easier, I guess I felt fulfilled by doing all that." When asked if he was suffering in any way presently, Mr. Kelch replied:

Mr. Kelch: I suffer her absence, that's what I suffer and that will be suffering until death.
Interviewer: How would you define suffering?
Mr. Kelch: To do without something you feel you need.
Interviewer: That's emotionally, physically?
Mr. Kelch: Emotional more than physical because I have, well I have a roof over my head and food in the refrigerator. But I don't have her. So it's emotional or psychological suffering that is with you every day.

To Mr. Kelch, suffering was not an easily described mental or physical pain, but the lack of something needed for well-being: his wife's presence. This definition of suffering is reminiscent of Augustine's definition of evil as the absence of the good. It was difficult for Mr. Kelch to restart his life with this integral part of himself missing. After he retired, he kept up with university interests and continued to visit former colleagues and students. These activities, however, could not assuage his grief.

Research has shown that the sequences or stages in grieving are widely disputed as to their generalizability. That is, there is no fixed amount of time that a person ought to mourn or conclude mourning. Yet Mr. Kelch showed a complicated grief that extended his suffering (Shear, 2012). After 17 years of bereavement, "suffering his wife's absence" remained acute and intense. The reality of her death beset him anew each day. Daily goals, purposes, or joys lacked the power to provide him with a larger purpose for living. The loss of Beverly caused *him* to feel diminished.

When asked what the word "suffering" meant to him, Mr. Wilson, who was introduced in the previous chapter, described his wife during her final stage of dementia.

> The last 5 years she stopped talking completely; (pause) didn't talk at all. She would stare at me, and occasionally she would smile. I loved to see her. But I don't know if she knew me. It's hard to tell.

Mr. Wilson witnessed his wife becoming locked within her dementia, unable to communicate or, at times, to recognize him. Unless experienced, it is hard to imagine the sense of loss that occurs when a loved one loses cognizance of all that she had previously remembered and valued, yet remains alive. Despite doubting "that she knew me," Mr. Wilson "loved to see" his wife, revealing that her very existence remained invaluable to him. He described their daily routine.

> I'd get up in the morning and bathe her and feed her 'cause she couldn't feed herself. Then I'd get her dressed and if it was a nice day I'd bring her downstairs and take her out around the neighborhood in the wheelchair. If it was bad weather, I'd put her in the den in the easy chair, play some music, or I'd put the TV on but I don't think she looked at it. Then I'd feed her lunch. Later, I'd make dinner. When she got tired, I'd take her upstairs and put her to bed. If she soiled herself, I'd clean her. And I had to empty the catheter and make sure it was clean.

The entire day was consumed by tasks of caregiving, which Mr. Wilson clarified had been

> . . . my choice. I wanted to make sure she was taken care of by me. To be honest with you, I just feel blessed that God gave me the strength to do it. I didn't want her to go to no nursing home (crying).

Caring for his wife at home in her final illness became an immeasurable gift for Mr. Wilson. When asked about an experience of suffering, Mr. Wilson recalled how careful he had been when moving or repositioning his wife. Despite this, accidents occurred.

> Sometimes, to give her a bath, I'd lift her and put her in the tub, and one time I slipped and she slipped and fell and hurt herself. I really felt bad. I felt guilty about that.

During the interview Mr. Wilson showed pictures the couple took while traveling to track meets. The photos offered evidence of his wife's personality and their joyful times together. He shook his head and handed the interviewer a snapshot that showed two smiling couples.

> I did a lot of traveling. This is my wife and I, and this is my good buddy with his wife. They passed away down in Florida. We were a tight group. We traveled all over the US. The problem when I look at this is that I'm the last person standing.

Although Mr. Wilson remained active as a coach, he is "the last man standing" in a group of his peers. Many men reported that they had lost treasured friends. They described this as a loss of the critical "resources" in their lives. When asked to describe a period of time during which he suffered, Mr. Wilson replied, "Well the best way to answer that is when my wife passed away. 'Cause she died here in the house. That took me a good while."

Mr. Wilson also talked about Mercedes's children, whom he described throughout the interview as "my" or "our" children. "My oldest, Gail, now when I go away on a track meet, to this very day she checks on me. She makes sure I let her know where I'm going." Still, he recognized that after Mercedes's death the children had difficulty "coming home."

> For a while they didn't come around at all. They couldn't stand to come here knowing that Mercedes is not here. I told them I understood. I said, "Come over when you're ready. The door is always open. But I understand, you know, your mother's not here anymore." This was when she first passed. Now they feel a little more at ease. Every Christmas Eve we get together with the grandkids and the great grandkids and we have Christmas Eve dinner and that's the only time we ever eat in here (dining room).

The ramp that was built for Mercedes during her illness remained in place, along with the deck on which she sat in her wheelchair. Their home provided a setting for Mr. Wilson to carry out rituals he performed to honor her, such as turning on the Christmas lights on her birthday. It also offered a background for Mr. Wilson to continue their narrative as a couple. In this ongoing story, he referred to the importance of lasting relationships, such as with Mercedes' children and his siblings, when suffering through loss. Hayslip and Peveto (2005) stated that the "how and when" (accident, illness, age) of a family member's death renders grief and mourning unique for each family member. Most of our respondents reported that the quality of their prior relationship with the care recipient was crucial in how they responded to being the primary caregiver as well as to how they mourned her.

The men interviewed gave care to their loved ones over years and even decades of their lives. When the care recipient passed they lost an important life role—whether they called themselves "caregiver," "needed husband," or "devoted son."

In describing an experience of suffering related to caregiving, Mr. Gilmore remembered Donna's fervent attempt to form words to communicate with relatives or friends. He articulated her distress at being "voiceless" in a gathering where conversation flowed. He described suffering this way: "Donna can't talk like you and I. And I'm watching her. So we are both suffering."

Interestingly, when asked how he would define suffering, Mr. Gilmore again spoke again of being voiceless—but in a larger political and social arena. He returned us to the question we asked at the beginning of this chapter—whether, when asked about experiences of suffering, men would describe suffering in a personal context, as experiences endured on a larger stage, or both. Mr. Gilmore talked about his service in the Vietnam War, over 40 years previously.

> Being Afro-American in America—we've gone through things others haven't. Like in Vietnam, we're fighting there and we're supposed to be treated equally, but we're being prejudiced against. They didn't want to serve us in the [social] clubs. I'm sacrificing my life, but if I want a beer, I'm treated secondhand. They go to the White folks' table and smile; you come serve us now and then. That pissed me off and I snapped a couple times. I was sacrificing my life. It affected me, it affected me. I could write a book.

In Vietnam, Mr. Gilmore voiced his displeasure, but without results. Both situations—his wife's aphasia and his inability to be heard in the social clubs in Vietnam—disclosed the frustration of feeling severed from the larger group. Donna could not put her thoughts into words, whereas Mr. Gilmore had words but no listeners.

In this case, "voicelessness" is the common theme of suffering for Mr. Gilmore. Whether it was occasioned by illness in the smaller world of family or the discriminatory mores of the larger world, it caused a sense of disconnection and diminishment of the person.

When asked about personal experiences of suffering, Mr. Davis did not talk about his wife for whom he was the primary caregiver but about the long-term illness and death of his mother, who had been hospitalized with an inoperable tumor when Mr. Davis was a young teen. Her entire "left side" was paralyzed. Persons who were unable to be cared for by family, who were without funds, and who had a disabling disease were placed in an extended care section of a local hospital. She resided there for over 30 years.

Mr. Davis: My mother stayed in the Mills Building in Philadelphia General Hospital and that's where she passed. That's where people are put who have no family. It's like a throw-away section. Ah, because people who couldn't afford to go home, they kept them there. They got the minimum amount of care. Throw-away care, I called it. But you can't afford to do anything about it. Later, when I was in the service I would visit her. Years after that I'd take my son to visit her.

Mr. Davis reported that his story of suffering began at age 13. He saw his ill mother placed in the nursing home section of a hospital for the indigent. It is hard to imagine him as a child and young adult who knows he does not have the ability, authority, or resources to change the situation.

Interviewer: What was that like for you?
Mr. Davis: Well, I was there at her bed when she passed and she kept calling me and calling me. After about 10 minutes, my wife said, "You have to let her go." 'Cause every time I would grab hold of her hand and she would say my name, and I would say, "Mom, mom, mom," and it seemed like she would come back. My wife said, "You have to let her go," and I let go. Finally she expired. It was tough. (Pause) It was very difficult because . . . (Pause) once I had a home I wanted to bring her home and take care of her. But then my wife, it wouldn't have been fair to her. (Pause) I had to balance all the time.

Mr. Davis paused several times while recalling the decades his mother spent in "throw-away" care. At that time worry about his invalid mother, responsibility for an ill wife, as well as parenthood and the demands of work were overwhelming. Unfortunately, his stress remained unremediated by familial or financial resources.

When asked to define "suffering," however, Mr. Davis, like Mr. Gilmore, recalled the suffering that came in the larger world of the 1940s. He recalled the racially charged atmosphere of Philadelphia when he returned home from World War II.

> I came back from the military in 1946, but we couldn't get jobs. And the housing situation was equally terrible. They [African-American men] had a riot in Philadelphia about [not being permitted to operate] the trolley cars and President Roosevelt called in the National Guards and they were on every trolley, sitting in front with fixed bayonets. They [Philadelphia Transportation

> Company] finally relented and hired one or two of us, but we weren't welcomed. Some people wouldn't get on the trolley if you were the conductor. Those are the scenarios that we overcame. That's what's instilled in me to do better because we were looked down on. Say, if we sat on the trolley they would get up—wouldn't sit next to you. As if you were a diseased person.

Mr. Davis painted a picture of a city and country divided by inequality for African Americans. African-American men who were soldiers during the wars in which our older respondents served—World War II, the Korean War, and the Vietnam War—expected that service overseas would change their status as citizens when they returned (Black, 2016). This did not materialize. Over 20 years later, Mr. Gilmore, despite being drafted into the "fully integrated" Vietnam War, realized that integration under the law was distinct from the manner in which he and other African-American soldiers had been treated in Vietnam, and thus distinct from the intention in men's hearts.

MR. BILL ABBOTT

We now introduce Mr. Bill Abbott, an 82-year old man who has cared for his wife Charlotte for over 25 years. The interviewer was welcomed into the couple's West Philadelphia apartment. Throughout his interview, Mr. Abbott articulated the insidious nature of oppression, that is, persons who have been "long suffering" in waiting for justice or equality may eventually accept suffering as their lot in life. Mr. Abbott witnessed the "tremendous amount of suffering" that assails persons of poverty in all ethnicities. The trickle-down feature of suffering shows its maze-like quality; it is difficult to find a first cause for suffering, or an exit from it. Mr. Abbott, in his longtime work in social services, spoke about the motivation of some persons to paint a person or a group as "less than" so their own group might seem "better than." Mr. Abbott gave a concrete example of our "places on the life boat" from the history of his community.

> I didn't distinguish myself as an African-American father until I got really engrossed in the civil rights movement. I just thought I was a parent. Then I started looking at things like education for my kids. (Pause) I even saw a difference in where we could go on vacation. When I used to take my kids to Atlantic City, which was the only beach I knew, there was a two-block area where Blacks stayed on Missouri Avenue and the boardwalk. You saw the same people in Atlantic City that you saw in Philly 'cause we were confined to that two-block area. That was a difficult time when we first started going to Atlantic City, trying to protect the kids.

When asked how this "two-block area" was separated from other stretches of the beach, he shook his head.

> The chains [that kept them in the two-block area] was inside them. Now later on this changed, but it didn't change. Oppression is something. Black people that went to Atlantic City didn't start going up and down the beach. Even without those chains on, they still confined themselves to what we called Chicken Bone Beach.

Despite ostensible freedom to "go up and down the beach," Black families protected their children by placing invisible boundaries around Chicken Bone Beach.

When returning to the subject of suffering in relation to caregiving, the interviewer asked Mr. Abbott if he thought his wife was presently suffering.

Mr. Abbott: Yes, mm, I think she is, particularly when she is cognizant, I think she realizes that she's suffering. I also think she's grateful for . . . things that everybody does for her without acknowledging it, you know? She isn't ever gonna give me a pat on the back, that won't ever happen.

Interviewer: How about with the children, does she give them a pat on the back?

Mr. Abbott: Well, she wasn't the pat-on-the-back type person to start with, that was not her forte. She appreciated what you done and in real good moments she would tell you that she appreciates me. But day to day, "You're a good guy" stuff, no. Whether she's ill or well, that was not forthcoming.

Interviewer: Would that matter if you would hear that from her?

Mr. Abbott: (Pause) I guess so. [If it were not forthcoming] it would not deter me from doing what I knew I had to do. Every once in a while she'll say something along those lines, and it'll feel really good.

Receiving or not receiving acknowledgment would not alter Mr. Abbott's caregiving but it would offer recompense. The interviewer then asked Mr. Abbott if he was suffering presently in his role as a caregiver. He responded:

Mr. Abbott: Oh, yeah. Oh, yeah.

Interviewer: Can you tell me about it?

Mr. Abbott: It was really suffering when she first got sick and I was the total caregiver because it inhibited me from going

> and doing things with organizations and teaching and stuff like that. That was a form of suffering for me, but I couldn't define it that way. I thought the only person suffering in an illness situation was the ill person. But caregiving taught me a new definition of suffering. I was emotionally suffering, and it was magnified because I felt stuck.

Mr. Abbott remarked that he held a narrow definition of suffering until he experienced the pain that came from a particular role in life—giving care to his wife as she endured a long-term illness. He continued with a thought that pervaded his entire interview.

> And I always felt I was suffering when it came to race relations, but I wouldn't define it like that years ago. The suffering drove me to deal with it in a fashion that I did.

We will return to Mr. Abbott later.

Not widely discussed in the caregiving literature is the care given to an individual who rejects the notion that she is being cared for. The care recipient may be in the early or midstage of dementia; may be experiencing paranoia, anxiety, and confusion. As Mr. Wilson described in an earlier chapter, he found his wife's handbags in strange places, such as a kitchen cupboard. She may not remember where everyday items are stored and feel that her thoughts are somehow disordered, but be unable to pinpoint her confusion as an illness or problem. She may not perceive that she needs care and adamantly, even angrily, denies it if suggested. The person who attempts to give care to this reluctant care recipient might be called "the hidden *within* the hidden among the hidden," highlighting the clandestine nature of this caregiving. In some cases, the caregiver and other family members also are reluctant to categorize the care recipient's behavior under the rubric of dementia, for various reasons. While conducting this research, there were several men with whom we spoke who wanted to describe their situation but did not want to be officially part of this study. One of the men, though, allowed us to report how he handled his dilemma.

Mr. M: You know, I swallow a lot.

Interviewer: How *do* you handle it?

Mr. M: I try to nurture the good part. Like, she has a wonderful sense of humor; we always laughed a lot. And she's got a good heart. She'll be the first to want to visit a friend in

> need. So you've got over 50 years of happy things in the back of your mind (tearing up). So this is all part of the marriage contract.

For Mr. M, "nurturing the good part" is a strategy for coping with the stress of being a secret caregiver. Mr. M. reported he knew several men "in the same situation."

> I have a buddy who has a similar problem. And he's disturbed about it, but he don't really want to talk about it. I told him, "Somewhere along the line us caregivers, especially male caregivers, need to get together and kinda hash out our problems to let us know that we're not in this thing alone."

In previous research suffering had been defined by several study respondents as [a feeling of being] "locked in, imprisoned, held captive" or perceiving "no way out" of painful circumstances. This definition seemed similar to what both Mr. and Mrs. M are enduring—he, because he fears the consequences of openly revealing his wife's dementia and she, because she is troubled by confused and disordered thoughts. Mr. M never used the word suffering to describe his tenuous situation. He viewed his "secret" caregiving as something he was "just supposed to do. It came with the territory." The "territory" was a marriage of 55 years that had produced three children and eight grandchildren.

He described his marriage as "mostly good." Although he was concerned about his wife's condition, he chose a silent way of handling her symptoms. He hid the work that he did for her, such as retrieving articles she had concealed and finishing tasks she would suddenly suspend. Although he knew that her symptoms would worsen and her condition deteriorate, he never raised the subject of her "forgetfulness" with her and felt that "things are okay, for now."

SUFFERING AS MOURNING IN CAREGIVING

Mourning in caregiving often occurred before the care recipient's death. It came with a diagnosis that the care recipient's disease could not be cured, such as Alzheimer's disease or related dementias, a chronic condition, or a disease in which the care recipient's mental and physical state either slowly or quickly deteriorates. Aspects of the care recipient's personhood, such as memory, a sense of humor, social interaction, and interest in activities, decline. Each loss in a care recipient's ability to remain "herself" usually engendered mourning in the caregiver.

Mourning also encompassed the physical loss of the loved one through death. The actual moment of death may seem sudden, no matter how expected or how relieved the caregiver felt due to the end of the care recipient's suffering. Death always carried a blow. In this section, we look at various types of mourning that accompany caregiving, and the ways they are experienced and expressed.

Mr. Brunson, mentioned previously, had given care to two wives before their deaths, and he mourned them after their passing. Although he was aware of the terminal nature of their illnesses, he reported that he felt shock when the moment of death occurred. "We were not prepared," Mr. Brunson said. "When the day comes, and we know it's coming, it's going to take a toll."

The "toll," as Mr. Brunson mentioned, was also unknown. Some men discussed illnesses that struck them after their wives had passed and their caregiving duties ended. Mr. Davis described being "paralyzed by sciatica" for weeks after his wife's demise. Mr. Abbott reported that he had suffered a mild stroke during his years of caregiving.

Many men commented on their prior belief that they would die before their wives. Most of the men were aware that African-American men have the shortest life expectancy when compared with European-American men and women of any color. For Mr. Kelch, outliving his wife was not only surprising but a continuing source of pain. We asked Mr. Kelch about what he sees when he looks at himself in the mirror.

Mr. Kelch: I'm shocked. Sometimes I'm shocked and I have to laugh because the eyes looking back at me are not the same eyes that they once were. (laughter). Oh, man.

Interviewer: When you look inside yourself, what do you see?

Mr. Kelch: I see a poor old man (laughs). My father used to say, "I'm just a poor old man, son, just a poor, old man. And I would say, "Now why would he say that?" And I've reached the point where I say, "I'm just a poor, old man."

We suggest that in both of Mr. Kelch's comments, along with mourning Beverly, he is mourning his former "self" perhaps as he was when Beverly was alive.

We asked Mr. Abbott if he mourned for his wife "as she used to be." There was no hesitation in his answer.

Mr. Abbott: Every day. Every time I look at her lying there when she's out of it. Like she had a bad night last night.

Interviewer: What does a bad night mean?

Mr. Abbott: It means she talks out of her head all night long.

Interviewer: So you hear her?

Mr. Abbott: Well, I did when she was more mobile because we would put her in that lounge chair and we would think that she would be comfortable for the rest of the night. But in the middle of the night she would get up and try to walk and couldn't walk and go right down. It led us to a lot of resources of which Micah (friend and neighbor) was one, 'til I realized he was sick his self. I said, "I got to stop calling on him." I started getting self-conscious about that. But we found out that if she does fall, we can call 911 and the rescue squad will come pick her up off the floor for nothing.

The poignancy of Mr. Abbott's comment was that his wife's nighttime falls, an unnatural and frightening event for most families, became almost commonplace during this phase of Charlotte's illness. The many tasks of caregiving began to include calling family, neighbors, and 911 to "pick her up off the floor."

The interviewer asked Mr. Abbott if Charlotte's long-term illness brought to mind his own death, or "making transition," as many men called passing from this life to another. He thought a moment, then replied:

Mr. Abbott: I would like to leave the planet before two people. I would like to leave the planet before my sister and before Bud (best friend). I don't know what I would do. I don't know what it would do to me to watch them go home. I'm okay if Charlotte leaves me; I'm sort of anticipating that possibility anyway. But ah, Lena (sister) and Bud, that would trouble me. The other thing is if something was to happen to one of my children or grandchildren. But we don't have our druthers; it's not our call.

THE RELATIONSHIP BETWEEN SUFFERING AND CAREGIVING

Caregivers of impaired or demented elders realized at a point during the caregiving process that they were unable to halt the progression of their loved one's decline. Research has reported that a lack of control over aspects of the caregiving situation led caregivers to regain control by miniaturizing. That is, they focused on short units of time and organized each day or segments of a day into a manageable routine (Black et al., 2008).

In our African-American respondents, we *did not find* that caregivers experienced a loss of control over the press of the caregiving situations and the care recipient's decline. A consistent theme among the men was that they were doing what they had to do and what they expected of themselves. Prior studies have shown that suffering is often related to an individual's expectations in life (Black & Rubinstein, 2004). It is here that African-American men reached into their common history of handling hardship and their expectations about life. Based on family and cultural tradition, men expected and accepted that they would someday be providing home care for parents, wives, and siblings, if necessary, and that they must be "up to the task." They were proud of what they accomplished, for the most part alone. Most of the men reported that perseverance in caregiving yielded intangible gains, such as compassion. Mr. Stokes perceived that caregiving experiences

> . . . made me a better person, more sensitive and understanding. We have a tendency to get away from being sensitive to what is taking place on somebody else. Now I think about that.

Mr. Stokes's comment spoke to the realization that compassion and empathy, traditionally considered feminine attributes, were added to his panoply of traits and skills through caregiving. Gaining these characteristics was a significant aspect of development and growth in older age.

As mentioned previously, affective and instrumental acts of caregiving were built into the historical patterns of African-American family life (Dilworth-Anderson et al., 2004). Our respondents were born into a configuration of kinship that included biological and nonbiological kin who were significant in their biography. Men spoke of survival, as Mr. Colbert said, in a "foreign" larger world as contingent upon the support of the "smaller" world of family and community. A crucial aspect of support was to give hands-on care to the population in this smaller world.

For older husbands, the meaning of caregiving emerged from performing reciprocal care. They felt gratified by the labor of caregiving that many men considered repayment for wifely support and devotion to the family (Black et al., 2008).Through caregiving, the "married identity" the husband and wife shared as a couple was deepened and prolonged (Brandtstadter & Greve, 1994). Men related throughout the interview that caregiving was "part of life" and that most interpersonal experiences that involved love also involved suffering and resulted in growth (Yang, 2008). For example, Mr. Brunson found that his "real self"—the self that was "always true to his word"—emerged through devotion to his wives. Mr. Wilson exemplified maintenance of the marriage identity and the role of husband after his wife's death. Men said they believed it was crucial to show their children, especially sons, how men should behave as husbands.

The men who had cared or were caring for an elderly mother spoke similarly about reciprocal care. Mothers had fed, clothed, loved, and nurtured them as children. Caring for her in the present was "the least [they] could do."

We note that interview questions about suffering provided a venue for men to talk about suffering in any way they experienced it throughout their lives. When men discussed suffering in relation to caregiving, at least two additional conversations occurred: (1) they talked about the suffering their loved ones endured during illness or dementia. Although men grasped what the care recipient endured at the end stages of life, they also viewed, in their mind's eye, a panoramic view of the *sum of her life*, thus mitigating some of the suffering that marked her end. Also emerging from questions about suffering in caregiving were men's (2) recollections about incidents of suffering they experienced or witnessed, such as those that occurred in war or just after the war, for which they never found good, definitive, or justifiable answers, and which continued to vex them. That is, suffering was a lived experience that reflected personal biography and history, as well as micro- and macro-cultural interpretations (Black, 2006).

Through caregiving, men looked into the face of finitude and at a type of death they saw in the care recipient that occurred prior to physical death—a loss of relationship with the embodied self. Although Mr. Abbott, Mr. Davis, and Mr. Gilmore perceived a link between caregiving and suffering, most men *did not* view caregiving as an experience of suffering. The term "suffering" was used by them for other events, incidents, and experiences in life that disrupted one's sense of self or caused a person to feel "less than" in body, mind, and spirit.

We end this chapter by offering a quote by James Baldwin (1961), who spoke of the genius of Bessie Smith to sing about the "normalcy" of suffering in African-American lives:

> The first time I heard this record ("Back Water Blues," 1927) by Bessie Smith. What struck me was the fact that she was singing . . . about a disaster, which had almost killed her, and she accepted it and was going beyond it. The fantastic

> understatement in it. It is the way I want to write, you know. When she says, "My house fell down, and I can't live there no more"—it is a great (pause) a great sentence. A great achievement.

Our next chapter explores the strategies men used to cope with the hardships in caregiving, or struggles that result from enduring other negative life experiences. We examine the unique ways African-American men managed their difficulties in order to move forward in life.

CHAPTER 5

The Strategies of Coping in Suffering and Caregiving

An important aspect in the experience of suffering in general, and in relation to caregiving in particular, is how an individual manages, resolves, or copes with it. When men spoke about definitions, descriptions, or experiences of suffering, whether through caregiving or other circumstances, interviewers continued the conversation by asking, "How are you handling/how did you handle this period of life?" Most men had accumulated, throughout their lifetimes, a repertoire of strategies.

In their responses caregiving men expressed themselves uniquely as well as with commonalities that spanned the sample. Uniqueness spoke to each respondent's personal biography, present context, and inimitable experiences. Commonalities resonated with life events and incidents related to being an older African-American man at a particular place in time, and to the emotions and experiences that this cohort shared. That is, their common humanness was filtered through the qualities of their uniqueness as individuals.

In discovering how respondents coped with the hardships that attended caregiving, we looked to answers men gave in response to particular questions asked of them. In this section we name three coping strategies men used in managing the stress, burden, or suffering that accompanied caregiving, either during the caregiving period or after the loved one passed. The strategies we witnessed most often were (1) having goals, (2) sharing the power of the family story, and (3) maintaining friendships with African-American men. Although the strategies were not the sole mechanisms men used to cope with suffering from caregiving or any hardship, they were mentioned often enough for us to note them in this section.

HAVING GOALS

Retaining goals or creating new ones was a crucial strategy for men coping with the loss and stress inherent in caring for ill or impaired persons (Micka, 2006) As one respondent said, "Goals make you look forward; you don't get nowhere looking in the rearview mirror." Most men interviewed planned a future for themselves despite the illness or death of a loved one, even if the future meant "the rest of the day" or "the rest of my life." Goals could be simple (Mr. Stokes's hope "just to get up each morning") or complex (Mr. Gilmore's intention to bring "the races together.")

Mr. Brunson, who recently lost his second wife, Barbara, had a simple goal: to attend a class reunion in South Carolina and reconnect with a childhood friend. The more complex aspect of this goal was to "get past Barbara's death" with the friend's help. By returning to his childhood home, he hoped to establish a relationship with the "nice widow" who shares his history and re-establish continuity in a life disrupted by grief. His goal also revealed the happiness he enjoyed in marriage. "I just want to live life to the fullest," he explained. For Mr. Brunson the fullness of life includes "the love of a mate, a good woman."

When Mr. Stokes was asked about goals in life, he mentioned two. "Just to wake up in the morning and put one foot in front of the other" was the first. The other goal came to light while he was giving care to his mother and discerned his sensitivity to others' pain. "I want to try to be concerned about other people and their needs." He viewed strangers as persons placed in his path because they needed help.

Men's goals reflected their generativity. Their concern about children and grandchildren was augmented by working with young people in the community. Many of them continued to mentor or teach. Mr. Gross repeated his goal—"I wake up and I keep it moving." He explained:

> I'm still coaching and tutoring the student athletes and all that. I'm still involved with young people because (pause) I think because I didn't go to college that I owe that to them. I want all my kids (youngsters that he coaches and mentors) to go to college and I use all my influences. And I'm able to do things for others. That's important. So I don't have time to feel sorry

> for myself. You don't have time because the extension of yourself becomes the care of the needy in your family and anyone else outside that you think warrant that.

Although those who know Mr. Gross mentioned that his talent could have taken him to the professional level in basketball, he was unable to attend college and progress through the usual channels into the pros. He transformed any regret he felt by using his talent and resources to develop concrete expressions of generativity. He "extended" himself to the care of youngsters who were in need of his mentorship.

Like Mr. Gross, Mr. Wilson also continued to coach track at Gwynedd Mercy Academy.

Mr. Wilson: I coach girls' track and cross country. I'm getting ready for a championship meet. I think we should win it. Most of my kids are sophomores and freshman, and all are very talented. (Pause) When I told my doctor I was thinking of giving up coaching, he said to me, "Don't do that, Larry. You have to have something to occupy yourself." My coaching helped me out tremendously. The faculty and staff over at Gwynedd were very supportive. They knew my wife was sick 'cause many times I used to take her up to practice with me.

Interviewer: Even with the dementia?

Mr. Wilson: Oh, yeah. The track at Gwynedd is named after me. It's the Larry Wilson Track. I used to take her up there. One of the students wrote a beautiful article about how I had set a good example for the kids. How I would take my wife out of the car, put her in the wheelchair, take her to the starting line, and she would sit there while I practiced. Sometimes I would push her around the track.

Mr. Wilson's well-tended home and the Larry Wilson Track at the Academy were points of departure for his memories of Mercedes, anchors for the couple's biography, and the environments that elicited strong emotion. Their home and the eponymous Track are replete with signs and symbols of Mercedes's presence. Mr. Wilson himself became a symbol of marital devotion for those who know him, particularly the young women who run track at the Academy.

Mr. Gross and Mr. Wilson coached young people as a way of channeling their energy. They turned their many talents into mentoring—which became a source and outlet for their surplus of generativity.

POWER IN THE FAMILY STORY

Most respondents reported that their skills and strengths were gained through family, community, and church legacies, and polished through a lifetime of experiences in these settings. Mr. Colbert reached into his family history to show how men of his generation were raised.

> African-American men were raised to respect, be polite, be professional, be proud, do the best job you can do, and appreciate the position that you are in because this is about being able to make a living for my family, which was important in a foreign situation.

Mr. Colbert named his home setting and neighborhood as the learning ground—his experiences in this smaller world readied him for the "foreign situation" of the larger world. He recalled a popular movie that depicted how African-American men handled the daily tension that attended living in two worlds.

> African-American men remind me of Hoke (Morgan Freeman) in *Driving Miss Daisy*. When I saw that movie, I fell in love with it because I watched how Miss Daisy thought she had the power. She never had the power. Hoke had the power but never abused it.

The movie also evoked an image from his professional life in social work.

> I remember many years ago when you [interviewer] and I talked [about caregiving] to those deacons [who were caregiving husbands] at the church. All they wanted was the recognition that they care for their wives. That's all. They knew they gave good care and were proud of it. I think it's common in African-American men and I think it's unique in them because I think it's a continuation of how men head their families.

Mr. Colbert witnessed this leadership in his father. According to Mr. Colbert, his father put his own needs second to those of his wife and children, even to the detriment of himself. He embodied a sacrificial love. Mr. Colbert named his family as the root for his "way of being" in the world. No matter how few material resources the family possessed, there was always enough to make up "another plate." Mr. Colbert grew up to be instrumental in improving the lives of elders in his professional life.

Mr. Wayns continued his family story and how they dealt with hardship. He recalled that his father exemplified the value of "finding work and doing it well" at an early age.

> I have been blessed and I'm thankful. But this goes way back to my parents. One time I asked my Dad, "Dad, how did you raise twelve kids?" He said, "I did what I had to do." He got us all jobs. I worked at the fish market; my brother worked at the grocery store, and another one worked up at the toy store. You go on that avenue you see us running around. You might think we own all them places (laughter). My father would go in the stores and say, "My boys need work. Do you have a job for them? Let them sweep up; let them sort things; let them carry and load stuff." My father got all of us jobs.

His father's legacy was an ethic of hard work and responsibility. He recalled his father's funeral as a testimony to his life. "When he died, it was the biggest funeral they ever had at that church. My mom died 6 months and 9 days after my pop died. I think she grieved." Mr. Wayns's smaller world of family and community offered him the skills, endurance, and loyalty to flourish in the wider world.

Mr. Parker described his childhood, up until age 13, as idyllic. When asked what it was like growing up in the city, Mr. Parker laughed.

> Oh, fine. As a kid, I was never home. I was out in the street playing baseball (laughter). We played baseball 12 to 15 hours a day. See, there was nothing we needed as a kid or as a family. My father provided everything. There was three of us siblings, and as a kid, I had a candy store account. My father would go pay it (candy store account)every Friday when he got paid. I'd go in and get ice cream, candy, whatever we wanted, I'd buy it for us.

He recalled when everything changed.

> When my father got sick and he passed, all of that stopped. I was like 13 when he died. We went from one extreme to another (crying). I had to carry on for my family and that's why I went into the service at an early age, to help support my mother. I always felt like when my father passed, I felt like I was the man (crying). 'Cause my mother never worked and she had to go find a job. So when I got out of school, I felt I had to go to work.

The power of the family story lay in its retrospective view of the past as a training ground. Telling the family story offered men and their listeners a sweeping view of the past. They could clearly see and relate the twists and turning points of their lives and link them to their current characteristics as men and as caregivers. Mr. Parker's life was altered, over 60 years previously, when his father passed away. This change continued to wield power over him as he talked about it. The story created a significant theme in his life—that of assuming the role of "man in the family."

> What I learned in high school was really the underpinning for the rest of my life's work. That's what I'm doing now—what I learned there. I came out of the Navy in 1959, and I've been doing this ever since.

Mr. Parker's family story began with an idyllic childhood, changed direction after his father died, then settled on a permanent track when he took a mechanical engineering course in high school.

> You know, you can see from my age that I could have retired 10 years ago or 15. You know, I could have retired at 62, which was 13 years ago, but I am working because I want to work and I love what I'm doing. That's the way I've been all my life. I figured that I took a (pause) a turn in life from when I was younger and I was playing baseball because I knew at that time I was good enough to play with the pros. But my family situation changed and I had to go to work. I couldn't stay out there and keep playing baseball.

In a way, Mr. Parker's narrative was a coming of age tale. At 13, although very young, he recognized and accepted that it was time to put away childish things.

One powerful aspect of Mr. Gross's family story is its setting—the "hard times" he witnessed growing up—which he encapsulated into a vivid story about one Christmas in the late 1950s. The portrait he painted centered on his family's struggles in a period when many Americans were enjoying an upswing in prosperity. The story also showed that the constant threat of poverty in African-American men's families became an ongoing battle against despair.

> I went in the army in November of '57 and before Christmas they authorized a leave so I came home. I was the most upset when I saw how bad things were and there was nothing they could do. My mother and brother—they didn't have nothing. My dad wasn't working. How much can a guy do if you are cleaning bricks for a penny a brick? You know how many bricks you got to clean to get a five pound bag of white potatoes down on 9th Street? Now that's an emotional state if you ain't got money, that's a terrible state. Now if you don't have the hustling ability—a lot of guys don't have that hustle; they sit there and it might cause criminality. The emotional state of not having—you got to have an outlet for that. You can't say let's wait around on the turkey 'til January 3rd when I get

> paid. So that's an emotional state but you operated it. That's amazing to me, we did it. Not just us, but a whole lot of guys did it.

Mr. Gross referenced an important means of survival and skill in the African-American community: to hustle, which had several meanings. One was to work at several jobs at the same time. Because jobs that were open to African-American men were usually low-paying, most men worked two or three jobs to earn a living wage. In their parents' generation, as well as their own, it was not unusual for a man to work in the post office all day and hurry to a night job as caterer or delivery man. Mr. El mentioned that musicians often "hustled" by joining programs, such as the Standardized Patient Program at local Philadelphia hospitals. They simulated patients to allow students to practice history-taking and communication skills. Another meaning of hustle was to earn extra money on the streets by gambling with cards and craps. For many African-American men, hustling was essential to make or supplement income.

> So I said, "You bet there is going to be a Christmas in this house." I took to the street and I gambled and hustled. I bought my sister the first Black doll in a baby carriage they ever seen. I bought my brothers a train. I bought a Christmas tree. I put on a dinner for 18 people. When I came home, I sat in the chair and watched them decorate the tree, and it was the most rejoicing thing.

The grimness of poverty and want was replaced by a decorated tree, presents beneath, food enough for 18 people, and a sense of fullness within what previously had been a void. Mr. Gross's story resonated with the meaning of Christmas. Its power dwelled in the transformation of his home's message of hopelessness and want. He "hustled" to give his family the reality of hope and plenty.

The power of the family story in coping with suffering often resided in the manner in which each man produced his family portrait. For most men, his family of origin offered a safe circle of acceptance and trust. Home was where a model of caregiving took root. Men's stories integrated the self into a family unified by their history and goals, thus giving firm ground to each member's future. For a few respondents, illness, the early death of a father or abandonment by him, and poverty precluded the material resources that helped provide this "safe circle." Due to his parents' circumstances, it was Mr. Gross who redeemed the family story. By "hustling," he constructed the safe circle of home for his parents, thus alleviating their suffering with his ingenuity.

AFRICAN-AMERICAN MEN'S FRIENDSHIP

An important way for men to handle adversity in caregiving was friendship with other men. The reciprocal nature of friendship among African-American older men has been understudied in gerontological research and the aging literature. Yet the men interviewed for this study revealed friendship as a significant value and resource for them as men and as caregivers (Black, 2015; Black et al., 2011; Mattis et al., 2001). According to the men interviewed, the nature of male friendship was viewed as functional; that is, men were sources of practical information regarding healthcare, finances, politics, education, and jobs. These friendships were also viewed as affective and emotional. One man spoke with a best friend every day by phone. In this section we show how older African-American male caregivers reflected on their friendships with other men.

Mr. Abbott knew his friend "Bud" from the time they were both 15 years old and living in West Philadelphia. Although Mr. Abbott spoke of his upbringing as "different from Bud's," they were drawn to each other in youth through school, sports, and social activities. Their "busyness" throughout life took them in both similar and different directions. In the present stage of older age, they have come full circle in their relationship. Each is integrated into the other's life through roles of godfather to children, standing invitations to birthday and holiday celebrations at their homes and their children's homes. When asked to talk about this friendship, Mr. Abbott replied:

> It's a fact that we listen to each other and learn from each other. We've both been busy all our lives, so the time I'm spending with him now is precious to me for two reasons. It's not going to last nowhere near as long as it has; one of us is going to make transition (pass away). So that the times we have together—even our daily phone conversations—mean so much to me. I mean, we are on borrowed time already. And this is a man I can call on in hard times. You can always find friends that can deal with you in the good times. But when things begin to get me down, I always know I can call Bud and he will talk me through.

Mr. Abbott described the reciprocal friendship he shared with Bud as "what keeps me going." Later in the interview, Mr. Abbott stated: "I want to go (pass away) one day before Bud."

Mr. Wilson and Mr. Wayns, who are neighbors and friends, enjoyed mutual admiration for each other. Mr. Wilson described the night his wife, Mercedes, passed away.

> I had to call the nurse who was in charge at the time and she came and declared that Mercedes was gone. My kids came over right away. I called Charlie (Wayns) and he came immediately and ah, he gave me support. That's why I say he's just a beautiful, beautiful neighbor and friend. I couldn't ask for better.

Mr. Gilmore described the concern his tennis buddies, "the Hilton Head crew," showed him during stressful periods of caregiving. When the interviewer asked him if belonging to this group "gives him support," he replied:

> Oh, they are very supportive; they even gave me an award for being a caregiver—The Outstanding Individual. The captain, Milton Clark, he lets the group know what Eddie Gilmore does as a caregiver, and as far as giving back to society in general. A couple times I got so overwhelmed with taking care of the wife—they requested I come with them. When you are a caregiver, you get caught up in what you do for the spouse and he (caregiver) falls into bad health. They talked me into getting back to traveling to Hilton Head with them because I don't have to be in this by myself.

It was not solely being invited to come to Hilton Head that gave Mr. Gilmore support and respite, but how the group viewed him as a man—an "outstanding individual." His remarks disclosed the significance of peers' acknowledgment of his work *and* his value.

Mr. Abbot plans a similar weekend getaway several times a year with a male-only group. Although he no longer plays tennis, he looks forward to the camaraderie that he shares with the men. Although retired, Mr. Kelch continued to get together with former colleagues and students from the university where he taught.

COPING WITH CAREGIVING, COPING WITH LIFE

The coping strategies mentioned in this chapter illustrated respondents' methods of dealing on a larger scale with the hardship of life as an African-American man, and on a smaller scale with handling the everyday labor of caregiving. The men interviewed for this project expected to experience disappointments and sorrows throughout life. Indeed, they had endured experiences related to being an African-American man that left internal scars. A commonality in men's discussion of suffering included using personal strengths such as "being fortified by the suffering of ancestors" in order to look squarely at hardship and use internal capital to overcome it. In discussing this expectation of suffering in life, one respondent said philosophically with a smile, "Well, no one laughs his way through life."

Although each man had unique means to handle the stress of daily caregiving based on personal characteristics and interests, there were also commonalities among the men in describing the most draining aspects of caregiving, such as cleaning an incontinent care recipient or wondering what is in the mind of a wife or mother who "doesn't talk anymore" or "doesn't recognize you." In a sense, these caregiving sorrows could not be "managed." Instead, the men reported matter-of-factly, "You do what you have to do."

One commonality shared among the men was the "normalcy" of caregiving. When they married, they had cared for parents-in-law and even grandparents-in-law. Some of their care recipients experienced "Old Timers," as several men called the dementia that accompanied advanced old age. One respondent said, "We just knew this (caregiving) was going to be part of our lives. We took care of my mother-in-law. I shaved my father-in-law when he got old. I bathed him like he was a baby."

If giving care to extended family was "just normal," giving care to a wife was "part of the marriage contract," or in the case of sons caring for mothers, "just natural; she took care of me when I couldn't care for myself." Although some men's lives were disrupted by caregiving and its tasks (particularly if men were middle aged when caregiving began), men fit the scenario of an ill or demented wife or mother into the existing schema they held about life in general. Most men worked within the circumstances of the illness to provide the optimum care for the loved one. They preserved, to the best of their ability, the care recipient's personal traits and core values by telling stories about her or recounting her attributes. It was not unusual to hear the words, "It was an honor to be her caregiver," or "I grew from the experience of caregiving."

Mr. Stokes offered a practical response to some peoples' expectation that, with enough money hardship can be quickly dispatched.

> I met this fellow in the lottery place. He said what he would do for his church if he hit the lottery. I said, "If the church is waiting for you to help them, I hope their roof isn't leaking" (laughter). Then I said, "Did you wake up this morning? Did you put one foot in front of the other? Are you standing here talking to me?" He said, "Oh, yeah," to all of that." I said, "Well you hit the lottery." [To the interviewer] See, I am on a cane now and across the street is a cemetery. I'm blessed that I'm looking in and not out. If that's the case, we all hit the lottery.

We sensed that Mr. Stokes has told this story before and will tell it again. A story was often told as an example of how a man came to be who he was. It created a portrait of him rooted in a family of origin, a neighborhood, and a community. The power of the story lay in the respondent's prerogative of using his voice to reveal wisdom in age. The start of the journey in his family of origin, the schools he attended, and the mentors who guided him led to the person we interviewed in the sixth, seventh, or eighth decade of life. The family story, like caregiving itself, was developed, interpreted, and refined through the events of a lifetime. Goals, family stories, and male friendships were made or taught early in life and would continue as resources to be passed on to others until life's end.

In areas of research that investigate difficult life experiences, such as poverty, suffering, or caregiving, some respondents questioned the "why" of these difficult human situations. In this study, the question of why was asked very few times and usually in relation to the suffering of the care recipient; the caregiver never posed this question in relation to himself.

In examining the transcripts of our current group of caregivers, we were reminded of an elderly African-American spousal caregiver we spoke with several decades ago, who wept throughout the interview and at one point said, "I ask God why all the time. I say, 'God, why have you been so good to me?' " This man, obviously in distress, continued to believe that he lived a "charmed life" because he married the woman he loved over 50 years previously, had three children, and was able to care for her after a severe stroke disabled her.

In our next chapter, we will look at men's religious and spiritual belief systems. We will explore whether and how their religious or spiritual beliefs helped them handle the daily frustrations of caregiving and of life. We wondered if they would describe themselves as religious or spiritual and whether the beliefs they learned as children "still held" in an old age filled with the angst and uncertainty about aging, caregiving, and the future.

CHAPTER 6

African-American Men's Belief Systems

In this chapter we explore the relationship between caregiving and our African-American caregivers' belief systems. We also examine how African-American men's history informed their beliefs and their caregiving. Their practical approach to hardship placed the acts and emotions surrounding religious and spiritual beliefs, as well as caregiving, into a wide-ranging African-American history.

"A book about caregiving can't be written," one of our respondents said, "without some discussion of our spiritual life." Another respondent described caregiving as "soul work" and that caregiving "begins in the soul." When asked how he came to be his wife's primary caregiver, this respondent replied, "Caregiving begins the day you get married. You're practicing all your married life."

This is where faith and caregiving came together. The men's comments suggested that they linked family, caregiving, and religious or spiritual beliefs at the level of strong commitment: Practicing one's religion or spirituality and caring for another human being require a day by day, durable faith. We suggest that men's belief systems and their ability and willingness to give care to loved ones originated in their commitment to honor their history. The wherewithal to remain a believer or a caregiver was culled from the depths of that commitment.

The material in this chapter was gleaned from the following questions and responses regarding men's religiousness, spirituality, or belief system, although men's entire transcripts were studied in the chapter's development.

Would you describe yourself as a religious or spiritual person?
How do your religious or spiritual beliefs affect or help you with caregiving?
Do you believe in an afterlife? (If yes) What do you think it will be like?

In men's history, both distant and recent, the larger world imposed its laws, standards, worldview, indeed its reality on all persons' lives. It was in men's smaller world where African Americans held their secrets, i.e. the dangerous memory of what forbears and they themselves endured as African Americans (Gutierrez, 1988). Certain intangibles also were crucial to their survival. They are: (1) ancestors' fortitude; (2) family and community; (3) sacred and secular truths propagated by the Black church; (4) bequeathing this knowledge to the young; and (5) each man's personal belief about "doing the right thing" or "living the right way."

Most interviewees remarked that a belief system was significant as part of their family or ancestral inheritance, just as giving care to family and community was part of inherited values learned in childhood. Some men named their religion or spirituality as a resource for finding strength within the precariousness of the caregiving situation, for stability during the progression of the care recipient's illness or impairment, and for comfort during the end stage. Men also spoke of their belief system as offering hope for this life that they would remain well enough to care for their loved one, and trust that the next life would be a place or state where they would be reunited with loved ones as well as a place with "no more bad knees, no more bad teeth, and no more cancer," as one respondent said.

Most men interpreted religion and spirituality through "works"; that is, they privileged the ethical dimension of a belief system by accomplishing works of mercy—the practical and spiritual tasks that one person does for those in need. For example, several men discussed the compassion that fellow church members showed by staying with the care recipient when a caregiver needed short periods of respite, or visiting the caregiver after the loved one passed. Other men mentioned the prayers that fellow church members said for ailing loved ones during "dark days." Men often spoke of the Golden Rule in interviews as "the right way to be and act."

Mr. Wayns was asked if he thought of himself as a religious or spiritual person. He replied:

> I can only speak for myself on spiritual things. I could be off course, but there is a God upstairs. I've told my son what I believe: If you are having a problem, you can tell this person and that person or mom and pop. But instead, get on your knees with all sincerity and don't be playing around with sincereness.

> You pray to the Lord and he might not come when you want him to, but he will come.

These few words described Mr. Wayns's perception that the foundation of faith is an open-hearted relationship with God. At another point in the interview, Mr. Wayns reported that he viewed his "many life blessings"—from a foundation in the church to his ability to care for his wife at home—as emanating from his "simple life." He expressed that his greatest treasures were those he already possessed.

> I think the Lord has provided me with a wonderful life. I don't need nothing. The biggest thing I need is my health and strength, and my sound mind. I got my little house, my car, my truck. I tinker around.

Mr. Davis described "the Church" as his foundation for coping with the many painful life experiences, from "raising [him]self from age 13," to the dire situation regarding "lack of jobs and housing" after returning to Philadelphia from the war, to realizing his mother would live out her days in the indigent section of a Philadelphia hospital. When asked if his religious beliefs helped sustain him during the years of giving care to his wife, he replied:

> Oh, those times were terrible, but what we had in our community across America, in the north and south, we were always sustained by our church. Sunday was the one day you had relief. The pastor had a sermon that fortified you, carried you through the work week in whatever job you had—janitor, domestic, laborer, or caregiver. Most of us knew the rules to survive and we did not deviate from them. And when we saw trouble, we walked the other way.

Mr. Davis described the churches he attended as a youth and presently as thriving communities that physically, mentally, and spiritually shielded him, held him up, and kept him from coming apart. They were also *havens*, the loci of truth not only about spiritual matters but about a world laden with minefields that African Americans might trigger unwittingly. They were given guidelines at church for how to respond to racism *or* caregiving. Regarding caregiving, Mr. Davis stated that the church environment provided an impetus to "follow through on your sacrifices." For Mr. Davis, the practice of religion was linked to the lived experiences that occurred—good and bad—on neighborhood streets. To him, Black history of the recent or distant past, as well as the present, is an ongoing sacred history.

Mr. Kelch differentiated between religion and spirituality with this comment: "I definitely feel that there's a division between a religious and spiritual person."

Interviewer: What do you think you are?
Mr. Kelch: I tend to be more spiritual, and the older I get, I think the more I become that way.
Interviewer: So you think age has something to do with it?
Mr. Kelch: Age and experience and longevity. We've seen so many things for so long that we've become jaded. I think age is a definite factor that once you've been around the circus, nothing surprises you anymore. You know you could tell me almost anything and I would just say, yeah, yeah, yeah, that's the way it goes. So I do believe you have to have belief in a doctrine to keep a wonder and an awe of life.

Mr. Kelch's profound comments suggested that adherence to a religious doctrine, with its guidelines for approaching life's mysteries through faith, may elicit humility. Life's many questions, including the why of aging, loneliness, suffering, and death are unanswerable. Although Mr. Kelch said he believed in an afterlife, he cheerfully seemed stumped when asked to describe it.

> I don't know (laughs). I continue to believe in an afterlife and I have so many doubts and reservations but I continue to believe it. My real hope is that I will see Beverly again.

For many of the men we interviewed, the afterlife was thought to be a state or place of reunion. If such a place exists, Mr. Kelch hoped to regain what he most treasured in this life—his relationship with Beverly.

Mr. Moore reported that he "attended the Catholic Church on a regular basis." He reminisced, however, about his long-standing involvement with the Baptist Church he attended as a child.

> My dad raised us in the church. He (father) was a single parent. For all my life he had us in church every Sunday. I thought that was what you were supposed to do. I was brought up Baptist; I still go every Sunday. That was just the way we was brought up.

Although he changed denominations, Mr. Moore never strayed from the religious practices he learned as a child. His religion continued to provide him with positive experiences of belonging to a faith community and indelible rules about how people should behave toward each other. When asked what principles have guided his life, he responded:

Mr. Moore: For the most part the Golden Rule is basic. But it doesn't always happen. Ah, turn the other cheek, I don't really live by that, but, mmm.

Mr. Moore later stated that he was troubled by not knowing whether he had or had not been baptized. Because of this uncertainty, he sometimes felt inadequate to discuss religious or spiritual matters in the men's Bible study he attended.

> I hear the guys in Bible study class saying something about they are on their spiritual journey and they are already Catholics. So I want to say something, but I don't know how to say it in class to them. Maybe this has something to do with me not being baptized. See, I'm not sure if I been baptized.

This comment seemed to hold layers of meaning. Was Mr. Moore troubled by believing because he was not baptized he had not earned a spiritual base and therefore his opinions were not worthwhile? Or did he link not being baptized with not being equipped with the spiritual tools to understand Scripture and suitable words to express it to others? The interviewer suggested that Mr. Moore could learn the answer about his baptism by visiting the church office and asking to see his record. The interviewer then asked, "How does your faith in God help you with caregiving?"

Mr. Moore: I'm doing pretty good because every time I ask the Lord, "I'm catching the devil today," and ah, the next morning or the next couple of hours everything be done changed around.
Interviewer: Maybe you know more than you acknowledge?
Mr. Moore: You think so?
Interviewer: Well, a man that's not spiritual does not ask God for anything.
Mr. Moore: Well, I do ask him.
Interviewer: Do you believe in an afterlife?
Mr. Moore: I try not to even think about it. But I'm concerned about the waiting while I'm here. I'm not trying to go right now. I just hope I'm doing everything right that when I do go, it won't affect how I am going to spend—after I leave.

Interviewer: Do you think you've done your best?

Mr. Moore: No. (Pause). I don't know if I could have been a better dad, but I probably could have been a better husband. But not to the point of leaving.

Interviewer: What you're saying all seems to tie into a faith journey, it all ties in.

Mr. Moore: You think so? I'm going to be pondering this from now on.

Although Mr. Moore thought that the men in his Bible group were better prepared to express their opinions—because they had been baptized or because their familiarity with Scripture was greater—his discussion of faith with the interviewer was plain-spoken, rich, and heartfelt. He measured his spirituality by his actions and intentions, and perceived that he could have done "better" *or* "worse." His candid remarks showed a thoughtful assessment of his perceived "rights and wrongs." In his comments, he revealed the humility and "all sincereness" that Mr. Wayns thought to be necessary in prayer.

When the interviewer asked Mr. Parker if he belonged to a particular religious denomination, he replied:

> I'm Protestant, a Baptist. I believe in the Lord. I respect the preachers and when I go to the church I go for the Word, and not for the people that's there. So, Protestant, Baptist, yeah.

Mr. Parker described his wife as "very religious. She used to sing in the choir. I mean church was her life. 'Cause she could really sing." He depicted her "last day."

> My wife had already made her peace with the Lord. The morning that she passed, she spoke with all the kids. She called them in the room one at a time and talked to them. Whatever she said to them, she said to them. And I don't know to this day what it was. And I never asked because that was between them and their mother and the Lord.

Mr. Parker beautifully expressed how his wife "finished up" her time on earth. His account showed how he honored her wishes during the last year of her life and at her death. Her request was to enjoy a last visit with relatives and to die at home, both of which he helped her accomplish. When she said goodbye privately to each of their children and made peace with the Lord, Mr. Parker regarded these conversations as sacred. He neither inquired nor wanted to know what was said. His poignant testimonial showed his inherent reverence for the "other" loves in his wife's life.

Mr. Stokes perceived religion as different from a personal spirituality. He explained:

> You know there is a lot of people who are sincerely spiritual. But you won't see them in the church. The others are sitting up in front, but their mind is someplace else. They looking at Sister Brown to see what she's wearing. I think I'm both religious and spiritual, but I haven't always practiced my religion. Truth be known, I was really lazy.

Mr. Stokes bluntly assessed his weakness in relation to attending church. When asked whether he believed in a life after death, he shook his head.

Mr. Stokes: Not really 'cause I don't know enough about it. I don't know about how that actually works. I hear people say it, but I am not going to lie. I'm claiming ignorance because I don't know what they mean.

Interviewer: Well, one of the things they mean is do you think everything stops with death or that there are some things that transpire after death?

Mr. Stokes: Now that having been said, yes, I believe in that.

When the interviewer rephrased the question, Mr. Stokes offered a different response. Similar to Mr. Moore, Mr. Stokes realized he held an opinion about the subject of the afterlife when encouraged by the interviewer and asked in terms that were comprehensible to him.

When Mr. Gross was asked whether he perceived himself as a religious or spiritual person, he carefully and sometimes humorously distinguished between the two. He recalled the generations-old spirituality of African peoples.

> Well, from what my knowledge is, we (African Americans) are a spiritual people. We founded spiritual. To mess with religion is a little different. We have Protestants and they have the Evangelists and Apostolics, and we have Islam and Buddhism, and the Catholics. That's religion. But spirituality, we founded that as Black people. But when you come into this society, things is imposed on you. The question on the paper will say, "What is your religion?" I can put anything down because I went to a Baptist Church on Easter. Or whatever church. I was as Catholic as St Rita. But if you say I know what Hail Marys are, I'd tell you I'm White. Or maybe I play basketball for Allah at the Most Blessed Sacrament Church.

Mr. Gross revealed the contingent nature of being religious. According to him, religious doctrines may preach love of others and equality, but if you are African American, you may or may not be welcome, depending on your skills and whether a particular religious organization might benefit from including you.

Mr. Gross experienced this phenomenon of inclusion/exclusion first-hand. For him, "religion" had been a tool to access church and school teams with coaches who taught him the game of basketball. The religious label a person gave himself—whether Catholic, Jewish, Christian, or Muslim—*was* meaningful. It could welcome or oust a person from playing on the church's team. Mr. Gross's wide experience in the world of semiprofessional basketball taught him that a talented individual is a commodity. Nothing, however, could change how people felt about the color of his skin.

> When I am with five or six White people, they light up and go 'round the circle. When it gets to me, I puff then hand it to somebody and there's no one there but me (laughter). And they ain't bother to smoke it after me neither. You see what I'm saying? So spiritually you overcome everything. We founded spirituality. Black people are more spiritual than anybody else. So I am saying that spiritually as a Black man I should be all right. Beyond religion.

This profound comment resonated with 18th-century slave narratives. Mr. Gross believed in a spirituality that came alive in the sinews of African Americans. African spirituality existed beyond the religion of slave owners and the religion that sanctioned slavery. It was born in the hush arbors that African peoples created in a land they had not chosen; it found voice through songs of suffering, redemption, and eventual liberation (Sampson, 2015). According to Mr. Gross, the ineffable history of African-American suffering and religion formed a bond between African Americans that stretched across generations and superseded differences in religious beliefs.

Mr. Gross: I know I'm spiritual; you know you're spiritual. Do I really care whether you into Islam or not? No, you my friend.

Interviewer: Let me ask you this, do you believe in an afterlife?

Mr. Gross: No. No, I don't know nothing about it. I can't (pause). I have no evidence. Ah, let me tell you two examples. Father Devine is one of my heroes for what he's done for the people. Daddy Grace is one of my heroes, way back there in South Philly. Father Devine had businesses all over the city. Let people get their hair cut for a nickel. He had lunch hour for kids. They had a haven at 16th and Fitzwater, right? I'm saying that each one of them said they'll be back. They never showed. I stopped even worrying about them coming back (laughter). So why would I attach myself to my heroes that ain't never come back? (Pause) I hope I don't see them neither because I don't know where they are (laughter).

To Mr. Gross, religion was human-made and offered no proof for its doctrines about an afterlife. For him, it also granted little solace for the generations-old anguish of African Americans. Mr. Gross reminded the interviewer that Martin Luther King wanted his people to enjoy a portion of the harvest in *this world*.

> Let me tell you this—I was body-guarding Martin Luther King. While he was in New Orleans, he was at St. Joe's where he's going to speak. They had three or four thousand people there. So it's me and him and the poor people of New Orleans. And a guy threw a stick at him. I was getting ready to rush the guy and this was what he (MLK) said to me, "If you go over there, I think you should stay over there." I never went 'cause he meant it. That's part of the teaching model that he's got. He gets up on the stage and the people are out there. He gave his thing and people asked him questions and guess what he said? He said, "We got to stop worrying about what we gonna get when we get into heaven. We need some of them things on earth." I couldn't believe he said that.
>
> **Interviewer:** He made a lot of Black preachers mad with that.
>
> **Mr. Gross:** Yeah, getting a taste of the good life that's here on earth, that's what he said.

Mr. Gross witnessed Martin Luther King's desire for a this-worldly social justice, or a Black theology of liberation (Cone, 1970). In regard to an afterlife, Mr. Gross trusted the evidence of his senses, based his beliefs on the wide-ranging experiences of deprivation he witnessed, and his heroes' inability to "come back." Laced throughout his interviews was an inimitable and indomitable humor, which like a spiritual created in slavery, also seeped sorrow.

Some men, like Mr. Colbert, connected caregiving to an active or working spirituality. He described his experiences of giving care to his mother, after being asked how his spiritual beliefs affected his caregiving. He replied:

> I think it is a privilege to be a caregiver. When your spirit is in the right place, it's uplifting to care for someone. You can leave situations physically drained but spiritually very high. Sometimes you are just soaring because you have the opportunity to do it and do it right.

When asked, Mr. Colbert differentiated religion and spirituality. He related religion to the negative behavior he witnessed in some church members.

> Religious people can be scary. They can kick you out of heaven (laughter). Religious people, for the most part I think, are full of crap. I think religious people are ego-driven.

Mr. Colbert perceived spirituality, which he witnessed in his mother, to sharply contrast religiousness.

> Spiritual is demonstrated in the walk and the talk. My mom was a role model. She'd tell you in a minute, "I know where I'm going when I die. I ain't sweating it."

Still, Mr. Colbert witnessed present-day religion as a social phenomenon that has much to offer in terms of culture, custom, and practices.

> Now I enjoy the [religious] tradition. It's tremendous. I'm eager to see how it evolves to meet the needs of the next generations. I like the camaraderie. I like the ritualism; I like the music. But it's an institution that is separate from my spirituality.

Mr. Colbert perceived religion as a fluid institution that links the present to the past and current generations to earlier ones, all the while changing with the times. He recognized that religion must continue to be shaped by the current cultural zeitgeist or become obsolete. He perceived his own spirituality as an essence filled with the love and wisdom of those who have gone before, such as his mother, and that persists in shaping and animating him.

When asked, Mr. Abbot reported he was a practicing Presbyterian and had been a lifetime member of his church. "I was christened in that church at 1 year old." When asked if he continued to attend church regularly, he said, "Not anymore. Ah, Charlotte's health and my caregiving changed all that." Despite his faithfulness to the church he attended since infancy, Mr. Abbott was adamant about *not* defining himself as "religious."

Mr. Abbott: By no stretch of the imagination am I religious. And I'll never let one of them preachers destroy my faith. I've had too many blessings from God. I'm more now what I would define myself as eclectic spiritualist.

Interviewer: What does that mean to you?

Mr. Abbott: That means I understand the connection between God and man and man's ability to approach him individually. And it means appreciating other religions, so that I don't preach at all. I don't believe in my heart that Christians are the only ones that's gonna be in paradise. That's going to be based on your understanding that there is something greater than man and man's organizations. I believe that there is a heaven, and I've seen enough of God's wrath to believe that there's also the possibility of a hell.

In the vein of faith as "works," Mr. Abbott linked caregiving with spirituality. He noted that belief and trust in God are based in his sense of God's presence in the concreteness of the here and now. He enumerated God's practical blessings in relation to caregiving.

> God continues to send tremendous people into our life and we had to go through several caregivers to find the right blend. We have one now that is like a family member. She said, "We got to take Charlotte out more often now. We got to take more trips." You talk about a blessing. That woman is a blessing.

Despite the many blessings Mr. Abbott spoke of, his wife's suffering sometimes unsettled the strength of his faith.

> Sometimes she talks really loud. I say to myself, "I don't understand why." That's the whole issue of suffering. I don't know how or why God would put that on a good person like her. I don't understand it, but I guess that's not for us to understand. We are finite beings. So every once in a while my faith gets weak. I don't trust Him as much as I should after all He's brought me through. That's the human part of it, I guess. They sing a song in the Black Church and it goes something like "Trust and obey. There's no other way."

The tension between faith and suffering was the pivot of theodicy for Mr. Abbott. It turned as he struggled with witnessing his wife lose awareness of herself. She would often frighten him awake as she screamed out in the night against an unnamed terror only she perceived.

Unlike most of our caregiving men, Mr. Wilson reported that he did not see any difference between religion and spirituality. He added:

Mr. Wilson: But I never gave it any thought. I have always been a member of my church. It's now about 67 years. But that come back from my parents. My parents were Baptists, my dad was a trustee of the church.

Interviewer: The same church?

Mr. Wilson: Yes. My grandfather helped build the church. We have a new church now but the old church, my grandfather helped build it.

Interviewer: How do you think your religious or spiritual beliefs affected or helped you while you were taking care of Mercedes?

Mr. Wilson: I think the faith really helped me when she was sick. I used to take her to church even when she was sick. Sometimes I had to remove her because she started making noises. To be honest, she never really cursed until she got sick. We would be sitting in church and she'd start cursing. I thought, "Oh gosh, I need to get her out of here" (laughter).

For Mr. Wilson, religion and spirituality were intertwined. The church building itself was a symbol of his parents' and grandparents' legacy of faith. Both religion and spirituality were coiled within the edifice that his grandfather built and the longevity of the family's membership. He viewed the unchanging aspects of his religion, that is, its doctrine and guidelines, and the spirituality of his community as faithful helpmeets during his wife's illness and after her passing.

Mr. El, when asked about his religious and spiritual beliefs, replied: "I continue on a lifetime journey. My faith is Islam; my religion is music, and I worship Allah."

His thoughtful response linked his creativity, given by Allah, to the beauty and wonder he experienced in this world. His role was to interpret these experiences in the language of his music and art for others to see and hear.

When asked if he believed in an afterlife, Mr. Brunson answered definitively: "Yes, yes. It's going to be beautiful." He then recounted the admonition that Barbara, his second wife, made in her last days.

> When Barbara was in hospice, she said, "Horace, you got to do something about your teeth." I said, "Barbara right now you are my priority." So I put that on hold. Now mine (teeth) don't hurt, but they look ugly and I love to laugh. One time we went over this woman's house, and that sister can cook, oh child. She threw down. I said to her, "With this kind of cooking you ain't got a man yet?" She said, "This man liked me, but he had no teeth." So, yes, yes, the afterlife is going to be beautiful. There will be no knee pains, no cancer, no bad eyes, no bad teeth.

Because most men said they did not know what they would discover in an afterlife, they imagined, like Mr. Brunson, that the afterlife would be free of the pains and trials of this life. As Mr. Kelch mentioned, most of the men also hoped it would be the state or place of reunion with the persons they most loved on earth.

RELIGION, SPIRITUALITY, AND CAREGIVING

A personal belief system for African-American men growing up in the 1940s, 1950s, and 1960s came from various sources. A traditional religious legacy was inherited from men's family of origin, and it was salient in childhood memories of Sunday school, choir, or like Mr. Wilson, in the church building itself, which his grandfather helped build. Most of our respondents had internalized childhood religious beliefs, which remained the lens through which they prayed, worshipped, and developed a self- and worldview (Eisenhandler, 2003), such as Mr. Moore. Other men were mobilized culturally and socially by African-American World War II soldiers who faced discrimination in the war and returned to an America still steeped in discrimination. The stories veterans brought back, particularly about fighting "a war within a war" (Black & Thompson, 2012) propelled an incipient activism in our respondents that also created a parallel track of spirituality as an issue of human rights.

In a previous chapter we discussed African-American men's sense of self as ruptured by a "double consciousness" (Du Bois, 1903a). The period of the early 1960s in Black history also split men's religious and spiritual beliefs into a spirituality that was activated in civil rights demonstrations or protests. Issues of social justice, always a sphere of concern for "the least" in a society, became a visible sign of a liberation theology (Cone, 1970).

The civil rights movement, as a social protest movement, mounted numerous campaigns, marches, and protests to shine light on the ways African Americans were excluded from participating in city, state, and federal law- and decision-making processes. The movement sought to end Jim Crow laws that, from the 1880s into the 1960s, established the illogical mantra of separate but equal, and legally enforced segregation in a majority of American states (Wilmore, 1989). Black churches spoke of the movement as a holy crusade pressing the country to uphold the promise of equality that was written into the US Constitution. Clergy and civil rights leaders walked side by side during the Montgomery bus boycott, in the March on Washington, and when the Freedom Riders were attacked.

Bregman (2014) wrote that "when religion is working as it should, it is subversive and prophetic, and disruptive some of the time." In other words, religion should call current cultural, political, and social philosophies into question when they do not reflect love, mercy, equality, and justice. Many of our caregiving men mirrored this opinion. Their engagement in theological reflection, or reflection on their understanding of God, Allah, or a Higher Power, was integrated within their concerns in their micro and macro worlds, and particularly their acts of caregiving.

Most men retained some connection with their church of origin. Some men looked outside their religious community to find a sense of the sacred, as did Mr. Colbert, who found spiritual increase in giving care to his mother and imagined spiritual pain to be "an inability to pray." Other men, particularly those who spoke of the tension between suffering and faith, as did Mr. Abbott, wondered not only about the tendencies of "man" to hurt and demean others, but also about the intentions of organized religion, clergy persons, and persons who defined themselves as religious. Some of the men interviewed discussed hypocrisy in religion, perceiving that it had abandoned its responsibility to critique society's mores, to be prophetic, and to stand on the side of the poor, weak, and voiceless (Bregman, 2014).

Many men described personal spirituality as whatever is most authentic in themselves. Prayers said with "all sincereness," "caregiving causing the soul to soar," "finding solace in a church home while living in a foreign world," and the primeval trust that Mr. Gross's and Mr. Colbert's mothers sensed when their sons were with them were true expressions of spirituality.

The interrelatedness of religion and spirituality within our caregiving men was complex. For some of the men this relatedness meant maintaining the religious legacy of ancestors, whether by attending services, social activism, or finding "soul-soaring" moments in caregiving. For many of our respondents, spirituality was a lived experience framed by this paradox: Life's most precious gifts, such as the relationship with the loved one, became life's suffering when the loved one faced impairment, dementia, and the end of life. Thus, in older age, men recognized that life's gifts and life's suffering settled together close to the bone. The power of this juxtaposition was that it was, like the Word, living and active, sharper than any two-edged sword . . . as it judges the thoughts and purposes of the heart" (Hebrews 4:12, ISV).

In our next chapter, we will look at caregiving as a pilgrimage that at least two people, the caregiver and care recipient, travel together.

CHAPTER 7

Caregiving as Pilgrimage

In this chapter we look at caregiving as a pilgrimage that two people travel together. We do so by exploring the caregiving path of one of our respondents. We differentiate a pilgrimage from a journey because pilgrimages usually are made by more than one person and more often they are made by a family or community traveling reverently to a site of spiritual significance. The destination of a pilgrimage is usually a place steeped in cultural, religious, and spiritual meaning, such as the Ganges River, the Kaba in Mecca, or a Christian shrine where miracles have occurred. There are many such sites attached to most religious traditions. The pilgrims believe that reaching the destination confers spiritual blessings, such as an awakening of the spirit to wisdom or discernment, or a greater compassion for others. It is a shared path, the blessings that the pilgrimage confers are granted to all.

Several of our respondents talked about caregiving using the metaphors of travel. Mr. Brunson talked about his wives' illnesses as a "hard journey" that he traveled along with them. One respondent described caregiving as "a journey that my mom and I, really our whole family, are on together." We used the term "pilgrimage" in regard to men's journeys of caregiving with their loved ones to show the communal nature of caregiving as well as its nonmaterial aspect. As many men mentioned in their interviews, they perceived that blessings and graces came to them, often when unexpected and most needed, through the assistance of friends and neighbors during their "hard journey" with caregiving.

We also use the word "pilgrimage" to note the liminal aspect of time in caregiving. That is, during caregiving, particularly in the last stages of the care recipient's life, both caregiver and care recipient exist in a state of ambiguity and some disorientation. The caregiver may be mired within the work of caregiving, as well as the sorrow of impending loss; the care recipient may be mired in the pain of illness or confusion. Both seem to be on the threshold of another, unknown stage of life. Liminal time seems to mime a vestibule or holding tank. Persons who dwell in a liminal period may feel betwixt and between time and place. They cannot go backward and are uncertain what will occur on the other side.

As we explore the symbolism of caregiving as a pilgrimage, we focus on one participant, Mr. Abbott, who was the primary caregiver for his wife, Charlotte, for several decades. Although he and his wife began the pilgrimage together, only he was able to recount it. Although two people, the caregiver and care recipient, are traveling together, each eventually ends the journey alone.

We used Mr. Abbott's extensive narrative to explore the notions of caregiving as a pilgrimage for several reasons: (1) the extended number of years he gave care to his wife; (2) the varied illnesses she endured and how they affected her as a wife, mother, and care recipient; (3) Mr. Abbott's articulation, openness, and insight about his wife's illness and the physical, emotional, and spiritual toll the journey of illness and caregiving took on them; and (4) his mourning, before his wife's passing, for his gradual loss of Charlotte.

Mr. Abbott's narrative of caregiving is especially relevant to this chapter because the interview provided a forum for him to recount his caregiving pilgrimage as both traveling a path with his wife as well as "struggling along" (Desjarlais & Throop, 1997). Traveling a path infers a smooth route; any distractions or ruts on the route can be sidestepped. "Struggling along" depicts either thorny terrain or travelers' difficulty in attempting to move forward.

In his account, Mr. Abbott shared (1) awareness of changes in his health as he continued to give care; (2) the effects of stress in caregiving; (3) the nature and meaning of support by family, medical professionals, friends, or other caregivers while caregiving; and (4) an experience of mourning during caregiving, marking this period especially as liminal time.

When we asked Mr. Abbott how long he had been married, he replied: "Next week we'll be married 60 years." He smiled and compared his wife's talents to that of another "beloved woman" in his life.

> Charlotte (wife) is one of the smartest people I've ever known. The one person that was smarter than Charlotte in my eyes was my maternal grandmother who

> hadn't passed the third grade. But boy you could not fool her. She was the boss in our house growing up.

When asked what the word "smart" meant to him, Mr. Abbott said that it was having the ability

> . . . to navigate in a society that is particularly oppressive. They (grandmother and Charlotte) had intelligence about life that I've been hard to find. It's knowing how to survive in the environment you're in.

Mr. Abbott admired that his grandmother and Charlotte had an adaptive ability to function and thrive in a foreign or hostile milieu. In explosive or exploitive situations, they "did not get rattled but held their own." He added that they were able to interpret nonverbal cues and double-edged comments, and to bring passion into a discussion without "ever speaking above a whisper."

Charlotte endured several illnesses during the past two decades. During this period, Mr. Abbott reported that both of them underwent emotional, mental, and physical changes. After a sudden fall, she was diagnosed with diabetes and other illnesses, and endured the debilitating side effects of prescribed medicines. At the same time, Mr. Abbott was moving from late middle age into older age and felt weakened by caregiving duties and his incipient illnesses. He also began to mourn the decline of Charlotte's health and cognitive awareness, his own health, and the marital roles (spouses, lovers, parents, social activists) that became altered through Charlotte's illness. At the same time Mr. Abbott had to reconstruct his role within the marriage and rescript their lives together. His story of caregiving was a concise, but not linear microcosm of the macrocosm of African-American men giving care to loved ones.

Mr. Abbot was 82 years old at the time of his first interview. He remained a sought-after lecturer on older African-American men's issues. He summed up the intricacies of presently giving a talk about this topic.

> I'm a motivational speaker. But at 82, I'm contemplating full retirement. This is why: it's the anxiety that it takes to do the speaking. I never used to be nervous about that. I put a lot of effort into planning a talk and as I do, the light bulb goes on somewhere and I just write. Now that light bulb don't go on as quick anymore. One problem is I'm not capable anymore. I realize to keep me from blabbing, I have to keep the period I give myself to talk always shorter.

Mr. Abbott's honesty about his ability to plan, clock, and carry out a lecture was coupled with wondering whether "people really listen anymore. You can say 'Amen!' all you want, but what do you do when you leave? Do you take an interest in learning about us (African-American older men) or changing our society?" Mr. Abbott's doubt about his ability to mobilize persons for causes of social justice was also linked to caregiving responsibilities.

> I have to put that (caregiving) first. It's getting hard. The thing is time—the time spent in researching what you're going to talk about, travel time, and time to give the presentation is looming larger because most of my work is done for nothing.

Mr. Abbott spoke of time as an entity that had become rigid and controlling. He also reported that he usually received no stipend for his speeches mainly because he was passionate about the cause: "getting the word out about the unrecognized worth and talent of a silent majority of older African-American men." He also wanted to dispel the negative stereotypes about them that are propagated in the media. Although he believed his topics remained critical, especially for African-American youth to hear, his worry about the time it takes to travel to and from a lecture site influenced whether he can take time away from Charlotte's care.

> And getting on roads like the Boulevard and I-95 is beginning to be questionable. I used to drive in the middle lane or the fast lane. Now I find myself driving more in the right-hand lane.

Driving in the "slower" lane became a metaphor for Mr. Abbott's life. Caregiving responsibilities, questions about audience interest, and awareness of "slowing down physically" converted his enthusiasm for lecturing into anxiety. When asked how long he had been giving care to his wife, he replied, "Twenty-five years in some form or another." When asked about the nature of his wife's care needs, he replied:

> Charlotte's had several operations in her lifetime—back operation, gall stones, all kinds of stuff and so she's toughed those situations out. But the first thing was over 20 years ago and I remember like it was yesterday. We were supposed to go to a wedding. She was getting ready and she fell down those last three steps in our old house. But we didn't know why she fell. Then in the exam they diagnosed her with diabetes. That's when we found that out.

When asked how he came to be his wife's primary caregiver, he shrugged:

> Well, it's like anything else. It sneaks up on you gradually. You are doing it without realizing you're doing it because it's minimal at the beginning. She

> instructed me on how to cook before she got to where (pause), and I learned a lot by watching her, too. The more I had to do, the more I did. But when she started with being incontinent, that was a brand-new ballgame for me. In our early marriage when the kids were infants, I didn't change no diapers. (Pause) So the first diaper I had to change was my wife's.

Mr. Abbott poignantly illustrated that the role—caregiver—he had assumed for Charlotte had engulfed his other roles as husband—lover, companion, and confidant. It was difficult to align those former roles with an extended level of care and nurturance. "I know that men are reluctant to deal with all that and incapable in a lot of instances." Mr. Abbott alluded to one of the most difficult aspects of caregiving—crossing the line between intimacy and giving total body care to an impaired wife. The private tasks of bathing and toileting are usually not shared with others beyond childhood or outside of serious illness, and they are often taken on by persons who are paid caregivers. This speaks to American cultural beliefs about the boundaries of the body, which must be crossed by the caregiver when the borders of the care recipient's body break down (Murphy, 1987).

We interrupt Mr. Abbott's caregiving narrative to provide further context to his life and to reveal his mindset about caregiving. Mr. Abbott, similar to other men interviewed, brought to caregiving a way of perceiving himself and the world around him. For most persons, this way of being usually began in childhood.

> I lived with my grandmother, my mother, father, younger sister, my mother's two sisters, and my cousin in a big three-story house. Everybody had space. Something happened, but I don't know what it was, but my father left when I was 6 years old. From that sixth year on there was no father figure in the house.

Mr. Abbott dismissed the negative stereotypes about female-headed households and described his home life as "very strong." "I understand the importance of having a man around. But I know it's possible for strong Black men to come out of a situation where there's only females." Despite a "happy" childhood, he described his early teenage years as a "bad" time. "Guys who had fathers in the home—that was a different ballgame. I knew the fathers weren't perfect; they had shortcomings. But they were there."

Mr. Abbott realized the importance of what he lacked, and sought guidance and mentorship from the fathers of friends. In 1949, after graduating from high school, a neighbor urged him to take an exam for a post office position. He was thrilled to be offered the job. "I thought that was the be all and end all. And a grown man's salary! I thought I'd be leaving there with a gold watch."

Mr. Abbott reported that he became a father and husband at age 22. He also talked about the "real" beginning of caregiving in a marriage.

> The journey of caregiving begins with a good marriage, and it starts earlier than what you realize. We started with children. But I looked at her (Charlotte's) mother and father, how they stayed together. And we both had a great love of children. Then there's the emotional and sexual piece. But the real glue is respect and love. And forgiveness, always forgiveness.

Charlotte eventually gave birth to three children, and the couple also raised a relative's child as their own. He named his work at the post office as "what really opened [his] eyes to life."

> When I first worked there, there was two Black supervisors. They kept it that way until after the Korean War. Some of those Black men graduated college and couldn't get a professional job. I was depressed a lot. I started getting closer to guys who were Second World War vets; I gravitated toward them because of this instinctive wanting to learn.

Due to the inherent unfairness in the post office environment, Mr. Abbott worked to gain pay and position equity for Black men. He admitted that he felt "satisfaction from agitating management." But he was not the only activist in the family. Charlotte worked with women's groups. "Both of us was always out doing things." Mr. Abbott's frustration with administration's refusal to advance more Black men to supervisory positions in the post office resulted in anger and aggressiveness in the work environment, and ultimately depression.

> I fell prey to the alcohol bottle and street life, and Charlotte had to put up with some crazy behavior. But I was blessed with a woman who was gonna stay the long haul, like me. So how I fought that depression was I became an aggressor. One guy said to me, "You got a big mouth, but you couldn't pass a college course." Another one said, "You ain't never going to amount to shit." Well, I took that as a challenge. But what that guy said stuck with me and gave me drive. I enrolled in Temple and found a new career in social work at age 37 with Charlotte's support. And I always understood what my role would be in terms of the community.

Mr. Abbott explained that the schools he attended as a child offered "good" foundational knowledge. Along with a zealous desire to learn, comfort with working "on the streets," strong identification with the poor, marginalized, and elderly, and snipes from coworkers about his ability and intellect propelled Mr. Abbott forward. He knew how he would use his credentials: He would challenge the larger system that created the structure of inequity for Black men, starting with the post office. His goal was to mobilize the workers.

We presented Mr. Abbott's back story to highlight the importance, when reporting on informal caregivers, of life context, to review the stresses and goals that compete for caregivers' attention, and to understand, in part, what drives them to give care to another. As previously mentioned, Mr. Abbott brought to caregiving a wealth of experience of working with African Americans of all ages. Likewise, his view of the smaller and larger world—through eyes that had experienced and witnessed discrimination, exclusion, and racism—and an advanced degree had equipped him to make changes in both worlds.

Mr. Abbott also clarified that because his father had left the family and its effect on him throughout life, he was, like Charlotte, committed to marriage "for the long haul." When asked to talk about the history of Charlotte's illnesses, Mr. Abbott began:

> It was with the onset of diabetes and the uncontrolled glucose readings, and her inability to change her eating habits, and smoking and all that stuff. And she loved her scotch, her and her girlfriend across the street. I think it was her inability to change her lifestyle. See, I was still working when she got the diabetes. I had a fear of what if I can't do this—take care of her? But I still put all my energy into work outside the home, and it didn't disrupt my life. So we went on until it got to where she was incapable of housework and I was incapable of doing it. The steps at that particular time had begun to bother me because once we was downstairs [and] we needed something. I'd have to run upstairs and vice versa. Then the washing machine was down in the basement. So it was hard on both of us. I don't think she liked that dependency. Privacy was an issue, so was cooking and caring for the house. Some of those things she took great pride in doing, bragging on her culinary expertise. The home was her domain.

Just as work was crucial to Mr. Abbott's sense of identity, running the home was critical to Charlotte's self-view. Mr. Abbott's initial fear after Charlotte's diagnosis was, "What if I can't do this?" He realized, when faced with taking on routine housekeeping tasks, that age, like caregiving, had sneaked up on him and that greater changes were imminent in their lives together.

> So we moved [into an apartment]; we were in that place about 5 years and she contracted a lung disease and we found out it was from mold, but it might have come from just sitting and not exercising.

Mr. Abbott's narrative was illuminating for what he did and did not say, and for some parallel aspects of the couple's pilgrimage on each of them. Downsizing after the diagnosis of lung disease was a new step in a series of moves the Abbotts made to keep pace with Charlotte's decline. Mr. Abbott fast-forwarded to when the instrumental aspects of her care began to interfere with his work outside the home and caused stress and sorrow.

> All her diagnoses hit hard, and I was by myself. Then we had to fight the, ah, the dementia. That's when the really hard work began, that was a few years ago. What the dementia did was—all of the things that I used to do were based on her cooperation. So with my help I could get her to stand up. She could still go to the bathroom and stuff like that. So that was the next thing we had to fight (pause).

Mr. Abbott believed that Charlotte's physical problems, such as retinopathy and neuropathy from diabetes and the fact that "she could not come and go like she wanted," deepened her dementia. He also revealed a difficult truth about primary caregiving. It is hard to *not* think of oneself as alone, despite family and community support, when the path of caregiving begins its steep decline.

> Just her sitting around when everybody else is busy doing something, myself included, with all my involvement in stuff. I was still teaching and there are rewards and punishments for that. Now that (teaching) kept me going, but she didn't have that and nobody [in the family] could sit there all day with her. So I think that isolation stemming from the physical [problems] impacted the dementia. It was another step down.

The interviewer imagined an impaired or demented elder brought to a gathering. Other guests greet them and serve them food. But with a limited ability for conversation with an impaired person, guests eventually mingle with those who *are* able to converse. Mr. Abbott narrated a portrait of isolation and stasis for Charlotte. Others seemed to be moving forward while the care recipient and the caregiver have few places to go within the shrinking boundaries of care recipient's illness.

A thought troubled Mr. Abbott: What if Charlotte went first? It was difficult for him to contemplate that his wife might predecease him. Like Mr. Kelch, Mr. Abbott did not imagine he would outlive his wife. At age 82, he believed that he had been "on borrowed time" for several years.

> And I've always labored under that fact that it would be okay because I would leave and she was stronger emotionally and spiritually than me. But when she got sick, I started to get scared 'cause—if it weren't for the kids now—she would have to be in a nursing home because I couldn't do it by myself. Now some days she's out of it and really incapable of cooperating when I tried to give her help. I would lift her from one chair—but I couldn't physically do it because my upper body strength has waned, too. Yeah, she wouldn't help me help her.

Charlotte was unable to "take up" some of her own weight when Mr. Abbott tried to move her. An accident in the shower precipitated the realization he needed professional help, and he changed their routine.

> Now Charlotte gets all baths right in the bed. No more standing up in the shower. I hit the floor one day in there. The last time I tried, she fought me about getting her into the bathtub. She pulled me down into the tub, and I hit my head on the tile wall. I looked like I was in the ring with Mohammed Ali. I was black and blue for a while. It went away and with it went my desire to try to manipulate her body anymore. But the aides do it now, right in the bed, and I watch them with amazement. They know how to do that.

Mr. Abbott believed there was a contributing factor in Charlotte's decline. She is the last surviving sibling in her family of origin; all nine of her brothers and sisters passed within the last 15 years. Research shows that the loss of close others during a period of poor health poses risks for further decline from existing disorders (Fiske, Wetherell, & Gatz, 2009).

After recounting the shower mishap, Mr. Abbott discussed the significance of having dependable, hands-on support from his children.

> My relationship with all my children is extremely good. I used to think at first the reason why they do so much with Charlotte and myself was based on their mother. Lately I'm beginning to appreciate they are trying to protect me because it'd be very difficult for them to take care of two people. And I am so thankful for my kids' spouses. They have supported us both physically and emotionally. They allow my children the freedom to come and help us, to stay all night long.

When Mr. Abbott was asked if he thought of himself as a caregiver, he replied:

> I do. And I differentiate that from a caretaker. I think a caretaker is a responsibility whether paid or unpaid, but a task that's been dropped on you; you don't do it

> out of love. Caregiving is an altogether different ballgame. You give care because you love a person and nothing else. You can't explain it any other way. It sneaks up on you, because most people, if they were told 5 years out—they might disappear. If they were told you are going to be cooking, cleaning, changing diapers in 5 years, a lot of people wouldn't make it because it's overwhelming.

This comment is reminiscent of Mr. Kelch's sense of awe at the duties he performed while caring for his wife in her last illness. Both men wondered how they would have responded if they knew, before actually giving care to their wives, what caregiving would entail.

An interesting aside is the numerous times Mr. Abbott used the phrase "it's a different ballgame" to describe the uncertainty of knowing what the next step in Charlotte's decline might be, along with added chores and their greater level of difficulty. This is an appropriate metaphor. Like a game with no time limit, no one knows when or how caregiving will end. When Mr. Abbott was asked if he and his wife were still able to talk together, he replied:

Mr. Abbott: No. It's all spontaneous and it comes and goes.
Interviewer: Are you surprised when it comes?
Mr. Abbott: Mm.
Interviewer: What does it feel like?
Mr. Abbott: It feels like the old Charlotte. It usually starts with her having something to say with me being involved in the street so much, my coming and going.

Charlotte's moments of lucidity and her conversations recalled the earlier days of their marriage. Mr. Abbott confessed that these were bittersweet moments. He acknowledged a certain joy that "the old Charlotte" returned even if for a moment. He then felt sorrow, knowing her lucidity would not last and fear that it may never recur. He described a sense of being betwixt and between—a familiar liminal state to many caregivers—on their pilgrimage of caregiving.

Mr. Abbott paused for a moment, as though acknowledging that although he had not necessarily expected illness and caregiving in older age, he had accepted it. "This time of life, older age, this was going to be the time of life when we have a couple dollars."

Interviewer: Do you think that anyone who is not a caregiver can understand your situation?
Mr. Abbott: Unequivocally no.

Interviewer: Oh, that was definite. Why do you say that?

Mr. Abbott: Because you don't understand what caregiving is until you go through it. I didn't and I'm looking at my own experience. I didn't understand, even though I was thrust into participating in some of my relatives' caregiving. I was ill-prepared when it was time to be the primary caregiver myself. And I've talked to a lot of guys who said that they didn't understand what that responsibility meant—what it was all about, how all encompassing it is, how the different professionals that you interface with impact on your life both positively and negatively in some instances. Every once in a while we get an egghead and, and you have to deal with that. But we've been blessed with some good ones, like Michelle, she realized from day one that it was my daughter she'd have to please, and now she's become like part of the family.

Mr. Abbott spoke to the various levels of ability, dedication, and knowledge in caregiving professionals, from doctors and social workers, to the aides who come to the home, and to those in charge of healthcare agencies who send out the caregiving aides. An important fact is that front-line workers are often poorly paid and turnover is frequent, leaving this job open to those without advanced skills. A broader issue is the fact that in the larger world those persons who do "emotion" work or "women's" work are viewed as "less than" in a technologically driven world (Ribeiro, Paul, & Nogueira, 2007; Stewart, 2008). Mr. Abbott clarified that it was not only aides who did not comprehend the significance of their work with the ill, the elderly, and those who care for them.

> I take myself as an example; I didn't have the respect for caregiving that I have now. When I was in charge of social workers, I sympathized with families and what they were going through, but empathy is a different story. Those in the social work profession and the medical profession and the religious community, until they go through that themselves, they don't really understand what it is to be a caregiver.

Mr. Abbott spoke about the all-consuming work of caregiving. It was not only the labor of physical tasks that consumed hours, but also the constant vigilance over the care recipient. The fact that there were few moments for alternative duties, plans, or thoughts made the time spent on caregiving seem especially liminal. There was no time and nowhere to be but in the small threshold of the present moment filled with caregiving chores waiting to be accomplished.

THE ELDER MALE CAREGIVER

A voluminous literature surrounds the well-being of the informal caregiver, which we addressed in Chapter One. Here we note how the Abbotts' pilgrimage of caregiving took another turn for Mr. Abbott while caring full time for Charlotte.

> The kids realized that full-time caregiving was going to impact me. I had a stroke in 2010. But it was never debilitating. I almost didn't lose a beat. One of the reasons I think is from being athletic. It kept my body in halfway decent shape and a blessing from God. But I was able to manage and get it under control. But even today my balance is waning. I don't know whether it's attributed to arthritis or diabetes, but I know I'm losing that balance. That's the reason the doctor don't want me to play tennis. He said, "You are too competitive. If the ball comes, you think you can run to it."

Like Mr. Gilmore mentioned earlier, Mr. Abbott's caregiving began when he was a middle-aged man working outside the home. Mr. Abbott was also involved in issues of social justice that "kept [him] in the streets." By the time he suffered a stroke in 2010 he was in his late seventies. Certainly, the years between age 60 and 85 chart multiple changes in mental and physical health, stamina, emotional well-being, and a sense of the future. Fortunately, Mr. Abbott spoke openly to his doctor, a geriatrician, who was also Charlotte's doctor.

> Her doctor, who's my primary care doctor, don't know what's keeping her alive because she's had all those scans and X-rays. His diagnosis is that she'll go down in the valley and she'll come back up and then she'll go down in the valley. As time goes on he said, "We are going to envision more of the valleys than the mountaintops."

Mr. Abbott paints a picture with his words. For anyone who has been a caregiver, one frequently hears the expression "new normal" during a debilitating illness. Each time an acute episode or event, such as a fall, occurs, or an added illness strikes, such as pneumonia, the care recipient's baseline health plummets.

> But he's [doctor] seen a whole lot of people that when they get to Charlotte's state it's all over. So he recommended we put her in hospice. For the last few months she's been on hospice and what we found out is you don't have to be almost dead to get hospice. Just the prognosis has to be that you are not going to get well.

When asked, "What was the best thing about being a caregiver, Mr. Abbott quickly replied:

Mr. Abbott: That's easy. The fact that I have not put her in a nursing home.

Interviewer: How about the worst thing?

Mr. Abbott: Realizing that you can't change much. As much as you long for the old ways, you can't bring them back. I can't make her walk. I can't lift her anymore. I can still cook for her. I think that's the one thing she'd say, "He's a pretty good cook." But she'd add, "I taught him everything he knows." (both laugh) That's the other part.

Interviewer: When you look at this journey of caregiving with Charlotte, how do you see it unfolding?

Mr. Abbott: Hmm . . . I ah, I have to say honestly I don't think she's going to get any better. I've resolved myself to that fact. Ah, I would like to see her go peacefully if I'm going to be alive when she goes. Nobody knows that. But ah, I have, ah, taught myself to believe that our ultimate (pause), both of our ultimate deaths—ah, will be a blessing whenever they come. And I say that based on her physical condition and mental condition and I say that in terms of ah, my, the societal condition of Black folks. It isn't ever gonna get any better in America. Some people are going to be able to make it, but the masses though are not going to avail themselves. That factor leads me to think I'll be glad when it comes time for me to leave this planet. I don't want to stay here too much longer with this nonsense. There is too much of it that I really don't understand. So that ah, I'm okay with leaving; I tell that to people all the time. They may not believe me but I am, so much so that I don't want any invasive treatment. My medical papers and all are in order. I don't want any aggressive treatment—life supports and all that stuff. I don't want none of that. When

> it's time to go, when the ticket is pulled, I am ready. I've done the best I could down here, I think.

Mr. Abbott's role as caregiver mimed other goals in his life. Although many would dispute this, he perceived that despite his best efforts, he had been unable to improve the images or refute the stereotypes of African-American men, or encourage the young to "keep up the struggle." Likewise, despite caring for Charlotte to the best of his ability, he perceived that Charlotte was close to the finish of their pilgrimage together. She would take the path to "making transition" alone.

The question of this chapter was: Are our elderly male caregivers "going along a way" with their care recipients, or are they simply "struggling along" as they accomplish the labor of caregiving?

Using the symbol of a pilgrimage, we witnessed that men seemed to both go along a way as well as struggle along in their caregiving. They traveled along the way of illness and decline with their loved one and gave her optimal care at each stage in her stasis or decline, despite the unpleasantness of tasks, and the fear of "how all this" would end. Those who cared for beloved wives also kept their marriage identity intact, despite the fact that some wives could not acknowledge their husbands or even recognize them (Black et al., 2008). Thus, our caregiving men also struggled along as they faced increasing powerlessness over the large issues of life, such as old age, illness, and the nearness of death.

CHAPTER 8

Addressing the Silence

African-American Men and Caregiving

We named the men interviewed for this book "the hidden among the hidden" due to their quiet profile in the realm of caregiving. The name "hidden" also was chosen because research on this group is sparse. Of course research on any subject is driven by particular concerns. Put simply, they are as follows: (1) society's interest in a particular subject or group of people, (2) the push of a particular interest group surrounding a subject or group, and (3) personal interest (such as our interest in the subject of African-American elder male caregivers). Calling this group "the hidden among the hidden" reflected the knowledge gap not only on African-American elder male caregivers, but the gap of knowledge about African-American elder men in any role that honored and affirmed their later years (Groce, 2002).

To construct a foundation for attempting to fill this gap in knowledge, we sought out experts—a group of African-American elder male caregivers—who discussed the concrete and existential aspects of giving care to an ill or impaired loved one. One fact that emerged through men's discourse was the dynamic interplay of culture and caregiving (Radley & Billig, 1996). The particular era in which men were born and raised (1930s to 1960s) shaped how they "did" caregiving. One man, when asked what makes an African-American caregiver different from caregivers of other ethnicities, said definitively, "Our history is implicated in all we do." Rootedness within their unique history forged a commitment to identify that history, particularly the fortitude of ancestors, the sacred and secular erudition of the Black Church, and the wisdom that caring for African-American others, whether kin or nonkin, assures survival as a group. At the core of this commitment to history was belief—in their eventual deliverance as a people by God, Allah, or a Higher Power, and the immediate need for all people to help God bring about this deliverance.

For African-American men, caregiving was crucial to this commitment. It provided a foundation for family and community, the "dangerous memory" of marginalized peoples, and current strength. It became not just a journey taken by the care recipient toward death but also a pilgrimage that at least two people took together, the caregiver and care recipient, usually with their children, and sometimes taking along an entire community. The loved one would not travel alone, at least until the last step. Each of our respondents narrated this theme of commitment during his narrative. Caregiving was not seen as unusual or uncommon; a customary comment about caregiving among the men was: "It is the right thing to do."

Each man also offered an individual narrative of caregiving that stitched the years from childhood to the present. Each man's theme within the narrative, although unique to his particular life circumstances, was also similar to other men's themes and seemed to be conceived in childhood. Themes consisted of a retrospective linking of events to form an unbroken chain of meaning to the present. The kernel of all themes was a situation that "turned" one's life, as Mr. Parker noted. He described his father's death, when Mr. Parker was 13 years old, as an event that made him "the man of the family," a role he assumed for his mother and siblings after his father died. This role also defined his caregiving actions and decisions concerning his wife. Mr. Abbott's father's abandonment of the family when Mr. Abbott was 6 years old shaped his desire throughout youth to find male role models, usually with friends' fathers. The lack of a father in childhood also molded his approach to marriage and children—he was in it "for the long haul" and he "would never leave the children." Mr. Wayns's theme linked the importance of his belief in hard work to his father's resolve in finding five sons after-school jobs. Mr. Colbert offered his father as an example of sacrificial married love—which became a true dying to self when he put the care of his wife and family before his own health.

While maneuvering in a "foreign" world, which is how Mr. Colbert defined the larger, White world, mothers and grandmothers were equally important. They gave their sons both love and discipline, buttressing them against the discriminatory and exclusionary environment their sons faced while growing into manhood. Mothers also bequeathed the example of a community investment in others, whether kin or nonkin. Mrs. Colbert always made an "extra plate" for neighbors, and Mr. Stokes recalled his mother checking all neighborhood funerals to "see if it was somebody she knew [in order] to pay her last respects."

QUALITATIVE RESEARCH

In any qualitative research study, what is not said in the interview is usually significant: Respondents often expressed meaning without words. Symbolic communications, such as facial expressions, a shifting of the body, pauses in the narrative, or silences are shared in place of words, but they are as symbolic as spoken language and as evocative. There are two topics we address here that may fit under a rubric of "communicated but not spoken." One topic deals with sexuality and the body; the other concerns the silent communication that occurs between members of the same group, whether ethnic, gender, or generation.

ISSUES OF THE BODY AND SEXUALITY

A sphere of hiddeness within men's discussion of caregiving was the issue of sexuality. During our interviews, we understood that this topic was pertinent and relatable to spousal caregiving, particularly while giving care to a physically or mentally impaired spouse. Yet it was rarely discussed in the literature and in our interviews. We chose not to ask specific questions regarding this topic for several reasons. One reason was to respect the privacy of caregivers' wives or the memory of their wives, as well as to shield grown children and grandchildren from viewing a public picture of their parents' intimate lives. Yet we wanted to welcome this topic if respondents wished to broach it. Therefore, the last question in our respondent interview guide (Appendix 1) asked: "Is there anything you would have liked me to ask you that I did not ask, or anything you would have liked to discuss that did not come up in our conversation?" A few times this query elicited the response, "Only if you turn off the tape." Other answers to this query advanced a discussion on subjects that had been on men's minds or that they wanted to "get off their chest." Some of the issues that our respondents touched upon were issues of companionship, affection, sexuality, and mourning those aspects of life as a caregiver. A few widowed men discussed dating. Mr. Brunson admitted that "having a mate" was one of life's greatest joys.

Although most of the men asked that their real names be used in this book because they were proud of their caregiving history as African-American men, they were also mindful of stereotypes that have accompanied the history of African-American males. These "myths" were a second reason that men were reluctant to speak about sexuality. A few respondents, however, brought up the danger of African-American myths, particularly those surrounding the African-American male body.

> Well, they're not myths exactly. They're lies. African-American men were used for breeding in slave times. Sexuality was their prowess. Now it's hard for that not to seep into your psyche. And you feel belittled for being boxed in that one dimension, or you feel you have to live up to that description.

Another man brought up the subject of the absence of sexual intercourse after his wife became cognitively impaired. Although he reported this to medical professionals, he said they were "no help." He broached the subject when he attended a "men-only" gathering at his local senior center. Men discussed the changing nature of intimacy while giving care to an ill or impaired wife. Some of the men found that kissing, hugging, cuddling, and fondling were expressions of intimacy that both partners enjoyed. Men viewed a men's forum run by "one of their own" as a safe place to swap concerns and express themselves to "those who could understand."

A different respondent related the experiences of an uncle who had served in World War II. African-American men's physical attributes were fodder for the myth he exposed.

> When he (uncle) was in England, someone brought him a pillow to sit on. See, there was this idea that Black men had tails. They brought him a pillow so he wouldn't hurt his legs by sitting on his tail.

This respondent showed the interviewer an email that his uncle wrote, many years later, regarding this incident. "That pillow," his uncle teased, "was life-saving. It allowed me to continue to walk for the rest of my life." His uncle referred to a stunning legend that followed African-American men throughout time. From ancient beliefs that saw blackness as evil, representing Black persons as devils became inevitable. In art, the stereotype of Satan was pictured with negroid features, satyr-like legs, a large penis, and a long rat-like tail. It was a short step from demonizing blackness by picturing Black men as animalistic and lustful to depicting the devil as a lecherous Black man with the characteristics of various animal species (Black, Groce, & Harmon, 2011).

Unfortunately, it was not only the dominant culture who believed the negatives about African-American men. One respondent admitted that when stereotypes were voiced by African Americans, "it hurt more." This man had entered college 20 years after the "traditional" young adult age and reported that he was asked by an older African-American woman about the subject of his college thesis. When he replied, "The positive contributions of African American men to society," the woman retorted, "They let you write a two-page thesis?" He described his reaction.

> See, now the Black community is my family. So when I heard something like this, it was more deleterious, and it perpetuated another myth about Black men—that they don't have the intelligence to make it in the world, or that they're lazy.

For this respondent, the effects of racism in the larger culture, particularly negative perceptions about African-American men, seeped into the views of some African-American women. Problems sown in slavery, such as the constructed portrait of Black men as physical specimens, breeders, the devil, animalistic, or lazy, were reiterated in many areas of Black life centuries later (Lipsyte, 1988).

COMMUNICATION

As we mentioned at the beginning of this book, an important characteristic of this book is its approach: Two African-American men qualitatively interviewed most of our African-American respondents. The first author interviewed three of the men.

African Americans viewed the method, analysis, and outcome of surveys or quantitative research methods as representing European-American standards and mistrusted their approach and results (Rexroth & Friedland, 2010). As noted earlier, if African-American men were to be included in a research study, they wanted their "opinions and history" to be taken into account. In our study, interviewers and interviewees shared the cultural, ethnic, and social backgrounds that drove the method, analysis, and background material of the study. Men's responses to certain questions, if asked by a White interviewer, might require follow-up questions for the interviewer's clarification. In contrast, an African-American interviewer of similar age, background, and role (caregiver) as the respondent might confuse or insult the respondent *by asking* follow-up questions. For example, when Mr. Colbert described the larger White world as "foreign," he expected the interviewer to understand his meaning. When Mr. Kelch mentioned, almost in passing, "the oppression [he] experienced," he perceived a shared knowledge about oppression with the interviewer. One of the most important aspects of a shared cultural and ethnic identity is what *does not need* to be said in a conversation. In any "smaller world," whether of family, group, ethnicity, or age, code words, bodily movements, and familiar verbal expressions communicate unspoken words.

In the qualitative, phenomenological approach to investigating the experience of caregiving, it was necessary to look at this phenomenon through our caregivers' eyes. As mentioned throughout this book, caregiving men had a pattern of interpretation about the larger public world and the smaller world of caregiving, and the "right way to be" in both worlds. We noted that men's pattern of interpretation held a double consciousness, or dual track of understanding, but perhaps it would be more precise to say that the men lived in two worlds for much of their lives. The macro public world made the laws, dictated the "truth" of events to media, and kept African Americans in the place the larger world determined. The micro family and community world was where reality lay in remembered history, shared experiences, discrimination, segregation, racism, and the evil that came in their wake. As much as possible, we attempted to do our research in this second, smaller world.

MEANING-MAKING

The attempt to make meaning of caregiving is shaped by a complex web of identity factors, such as family legacy and tradition, religious and spiritual beliefs, trust or lack of trust in the larger medical system and in local healthcare professionals, attributions of illness, beliefs about the "self" in dementia, and the principles that steer a personal morality of caregiving. As such, the questions that we asked caregivers were guided by an assumption that the meaning of caregiving occurs at the core of the individual, where a culture of caregiving, witnessed by the men while growing up, was internalized. Thus, giving care to another held moral and sacred connotations. Sensibilities of what is right or wrong, the meaning of commitment, and the value of "keeping your word" were as fundamental to caregiving as to living life.

NARRATIVE

We do not suggest that the caregiving narratives of 13 men delimit the African-American elder male caregiver or render this study as generalizable to the larger population of African-American men. The narratives however, like literature, do grant a perspective of reality. They offer a window onto a small, hidden section of our society—African-American male caregivers and their stories of caregiving that allowed us into their world. They were a inimitable source for understanding the nature of their experiences of caregiving while they also highlighted a history that shaped the necessity of caregiving. We cannot hear "the scream in the night" that wakes the caregiver out of sleep, but we can stand for a moment at the edge of that abyss, imagining with him what dark hole or endless expanse in the mind generated that scream. Their narratives *may* be generalized as a privileged insight into the world of African-American elder male caregiving.

The notion of generatiavity has expanded in the preceding decades. Rubinstein et al. (2014) noted that caring for elders is investing in one's origins. It actually places the self (in this case the caregiver) as the center in a triptych between the past and the future, in which all of the men have given or may give care to the other. Caregivers' children closely observed the honor given to the care recipient in the latter stages of life. As one caregiver said:

> "My life can't impact on anybody unless it's explained to them. We can't learn from anybody if we don't know our history, whether that's the history of African Americans in America or the history of us as caregivers."

One of the most important aspects in the fulfillment of this research was that our interviewers were African-American men. They highlighted the importance of researchers living, working, and giving care in the same culture as the respondents. The significance of an investigator being "recognizable" to the respondents, in age as well as ethnicity, contributed to the depth of the findings of this research.

We note that this book was not written solely for caregivers, care recipients, or professionals in the fields of social work, gerontology, or African-American studies. It was written because caregivers' narratives have the power to provoke empathy in the reader who perhaps is dissimilar to the caregiver in age, ethnicity, or role as caregiver, but learns from others' lives. We believe that the narratives of our caregiving men can broaden readers' moral imagination. They can witness a world in which care recipients are traveling toward the last stages of life. Caregivers' response is that they will travel with them on this pilgrimage as far as they are able.

FUTURE RESEARCH

We attempted to show the multidimensional complexity and integration of caregiving in men's lives. The significance of commitment to family and community in African-American history was an impetus for caregiving, for honoring a centuries-old belief system, and for merging a reverence for ancestors with a concern for the future of African-Americans.

The role of culture and belief systems in the past and present in shaping the dynamic experience of caregiving is a worthy area of exploration in future studies of caregiving. Likewise, a more expansive examination of the nature and meaning of caregiving among this cohort could clarify the issues important to male caregivers, along with how male caregivers culturally construct their life course before, during, and after caregiving. Interestingly, as the men in this study showed, the life course may have dual tracks for African-American caregiving men, reflecting the two worlds that men either discussed or inferred. Caregivers' responses to caregiving may be approached by exploring each caregiver's sense of commitment, which takes culture, religious and spiritual belief, communal history, recent and ancestral family, and kin and nonkin into account. For the men interviewed, this pattern of interpreting the world seemed to begin early in life.

Perhaps one of the most important questions in this book must come at its end. Will the children and grandchildren of our African-American caregivers fulfill a similar role as their fathers and grandfathers, that is as caregivers for kin or non-kin? Several of our respondents wondered about younger generations and worried that individualism might look more attractive than the communal history their fathers emulated, or that their sons and grandsons might believe there is no longer a need for the "struggle" to continue. Current events reveal that *all* people need to be aware and engaged in all other persons' struggles against divisiveness, exclusion, or separatism. As one of our respondents said pointedly and poignantly, "We can ill afford to be individualists in this society."

APPENDIX A

Resource Listing

We have included a list of national organizations that are important resources for caregivers, care recipients, and professionals. Although we have offered each national organization's address, phone number, and Web site, all organizations have area or local agencies. By calling the national agency, no matter what city or state you live in, you will be given an address, number, and Web site for the agency nearest you.

1. Agency for Healthcare Research and Quality Publications Clearinghouse
   PO Box 8547
   Silver Spring, MD 20907-8547
   1-800-358-9295 (toll-free)
   1-888-586-6340 (TDD/toll-free)
   www.ahrq.gov
2. American Cancer Society
   1-800-227-2345 (toll-free)
   1-866-228-4327 (TTY/toll-free)
   www.cancer.org
3. American Urological Association Foundation
   1000 Corporate Boulevard
   Linthicum, MD 21090
   1-800-828-7866 (toll-free)
   www.auafoundation.org
4. National Cancer Institute
   Cancer Information Service
   1-800-422-6237 (toll-free)
   1-800-332-8615 (TTY/toll-free)
   www.cancer.gov/prostate

5. National Kidney and Urological Diseases Information Clearinghouse
   3 Information Way
   Bethesda, MD 20892-3580
   1-800-891-5390 (toll-free)
   1-866-569-1162 (TTY/toll-free)
   www.kidney.niddk.nih.gov
6. National Institute on Aging
   Information Center
   PO Box 8057
   Gaithersburg, MD 20898-8057
   1-800-222-2225 (toll-free)
   1-800-222-4225 (TTY/toll-free)
   www.nia.nih.gov
   www.nia.nih.gov/Espanol
   National Library of Medicine
   www.nihseniorhealth.gov
7. American Heart Association
   7272 Greenville Avenue
   Dallas, TX 75231
   1-800-242-8721 (toll-free)
   www.heart.org
8. National Heart, Lung, and Blood Institute
   Health Information Center
   PO Box 30105
   Bethesda, MD 20824-0105
   1-301-592-8573
   www.nhlbi.nih.gov
9. National Library of Medicine MedlinePlus
   www.medlineplus.gov
10. American Association for Geriatric Psychiatry
    7910 Woodmont Avenue, Suite 1050
    Bethesda, MD 20814-3004
    1-301-654-7850
    www.aagponline.org
11. Depression and Bipolar Support Alliance
    730 North Franklin Street, Suite 501
    Chicago, IL 60654-7225
    1-800-826-3632 (toll-free)
    www.dbsalliance.org

12. National Alliance on Mental Illness
    3803 North Fairfax Drive, Suite 100
    Arlington, VA 22203
    1-800-950-6264 (toll-free)
    www.nami.org
13. National Institute on Mental Health
    6001 Executive Boulevard
    Room 6200, MSC 9663
    Bethesda, MD 20892-9663
    1-866-615-6464 (toll-free)
    1-866-415-8051 (TTY/toll-free)
    www.nimh.nih.gov
14. American Stroke Association
    7272 Greenville Avenue
    Dallas, TX 75231
    1-888-478-7653 (toll-free)
    1-888-474-8483 (toll-free, Spanish)
    www.strokeassociation.org
    National Stroke Association
    9707 East Easter Lane, Suite B
    Centennial, CO 80112
    1-800-787-6537 (toll-free)
    www.stoke.org
15. American Diabetes Association
    1701 North Beauegard Street
    Alexandria, VA 22311
    1-800-342-2383 (toll-free)
    www.diabetes.org
16. National Diabetes Education Program
    One Diabetes Way
    Bethesda, MD 20814-9692
    1-888-693-6337 (toll-free)
    www.ndep.nih.gov
17. National Diabetes Information Clearinghouse (NDIC)
    National Institute of Diabetes and Digestive and Kidney Diseases
    1 Information Way
    Bethesda, MD 20892-3560
    1-800-860-8747 (toll-free)
    1-866-569-1162 (TTY/toll-free)
    www.diabetes.niddk.nih.gov

18. American Association for Retired Persons (AARP)
    1-888-687-2277
    www.aarp.org
19. American Lung Association
    1301 Pennsylvania Ave, NW
    Suite 800
    Washington, DC 20004
    1-202-785-3355
    1-800-548-8252 (lung helpline, toll-free)
    www.lungsusa.org
20. Alzheimer's Association
    24/7 Helpline
    1-800-272-3900
21. Alzheimer's Disease Education and Referral Center
    PO Box 8250
    Silver Spring, MD 20907
    1-800-438-4380
22. Eldercare Locator
    (links seniors, families, and professionals with state and local area agencies on aging, along with other state and federal eldercare and senior service organizations)
    1-800-677-1116
    www.eldercare.gov
23. American Geriatrics Society
    40 Fulton Street, 18th floor
    New York, NY 10038
    1-212-308-1414
    www.healthinaging.org
24. Centers for Medicare and Medicaid Services
    7500 Security Boulevard
    Baltimore, MD 21244
    1-800-Medicare (toll-free)
    1-800-633-4227
    1-877-486-2048 (TTY/toll-free)
    www.medicare.gov

The organizations listed here and their local chapters can put you in touch with a support group. When thinking about accessing a site, it is important to remember that you are not alone. Many people are in similar positions. The only way we can know that services are available is to ask. This is a way to start.

APPENDIX B

Research Interview Guide

TIME 1 QUESTIONNAIRE

We are interested in talking to African-American older men who are or have been primary caregivers in their home, and who have been caring for someone for 2 years or more.

The first thing I'd like to do is ask you a few background questions about yourself.

How old are you?

What is your birthdate?

What is/was your occupation? The following questions on this page should read:

How would you rate your physical health right now?
Excellent Good Fair Poor

Why do you rate it that way?

How would you rate your emotional health right now?
Excellent Good Fair Poor

Why do you rate it that way?

What is your marital status? ______________________________

(if married)
How many years have you been married? ____________________

(If wife is deceased)
How many years were you married?________________________

What is/was your wife's name?______________________________

How did you meet her?

What was she like back then?
(Probe for mutual attraction, when he knew "she was the one."

Do you have children? Yes No
(circle correct answer)

(if yes) **How many?**

Can you name each one and where they live?
Name__________________________
Residence______________________
How often do you see?___________________

I'd like to ask you a few questions about being a parent.

What is it like to be an African-American father?

What is your favorite thing about being a parent?

How about your least favorite thing?

What is your relationship like with each of the children?

What is/was your wife's favorite thing about being a parent?

How about her least favorite?

(If wife is living) **What is your wife's current relationship like with the children?**

Tell me a little more about you. Where did you grow up? What was your family like? (probe for family qualities, siblings, friends, neighborhood)

Do you practice a particular religion?______________________________
(probe for how often attends services, participates in any church groups)

CAREGIVING

Now we are going to talk a little more about caregiving
How long have you been caring for ____________________?

What is his/her illness?

Can you describe him/her for me?

How has the illness affected his/her personality?

What were the first signs of his/her illness?

Did you notice this first or did someone else bring it to your attention?

How did you come to be the main person caring for him/her?

Some people, even though they do a lot for another person, don't call themselves a caregiver. Do you think of yourself as a caregiver?

When you were growing up, did you see your parents care for anybody in the home? (probe, what did respondent think about that; did he share in the caregiving responsibilities)

Let's talk about day-to-day life for you and (care recipient)__________
____

Can you describe a typical day for me?

What is your favorite time of the day? (Why?)

How about your least favorite? (Why?)

Can you tell me the best things about being a caregiver?

How about the worst?

As we mentioned, we are studying AA elder male caregivers like you because there has been so little written about the work they do. In fact, they are often called "hidden" caregivers.

In your own words, what does it mean to be an AA older man who is giving care to another person?

Why do you do it?

When we first started talking, you described your health as _______________. Can you tell me why?

Do any health problems stand in the way of doing things you want to do?
(Probe for any condition, how treated, coped with presently, and if it grows harder to cope with caregiving, or his own illness as time goes by)

How does caregiving affect your health? (probe for emotional and physical health)

____

Has your health had to take a backseat since being a caregiver?

Does your doctor know you are a caregiver? Do you talk with him/her about being a caregiver?

T2 QUESTIONNAIRE

Note: Bolded statements should be read out loud. Notes in ( ) are directions for interviewer.

I hope you know how much we appreciate your being a part of this study.

After we went over your answers from the first interview, we came up with a few follow-up questions.

(Use this space to write in follow up questions)

<u>Now we can start we some new questions:</u>

SUPPORT

Can you tell me about a person or people who are or have been particularly supportive of you as a caregiver?

Name ____________________ Type of support given ____________S

Are there people in your life who are not/have not been particularly supportive that you thought might be or wished they would be?
(Probe: Ask respondent to name the person, what kind of help they hoped for from the person, and what occurred)

Do you think anyone *<u>who is not</u>* a caregiver can understand your situation?

ISSUES OF CONTROL

Do you feel you have control over your life and the way it is going? (Why? Or why not?)

Thinking about your life, when have you felt most "in control" of your life?

Thinking about your life, when have you felt most "out of control" of your life? (probe for why he felt that way and how he handled it)

How about right now, in relation to caregiving, do you feel you are in control of the work you have to do? (probe for why or why not)

Tell me how you think this journey of caregiving will unfold?

ISSUES OF SUFFERING

Can you name one or two things that you regret about your life?

Sometimes we are hard on ourselves about things we did or did not do.

Do you think you are hard on yourself about some things? Can you tell me what?

Sometimes it is hard to forgive ourselves for things we did or did not do.

Do you think you are able to forgive yourself for anything you think you did wrong?

Would you describe yourself as suffering in any way presently?
How would you define suffering?

How about in the past, do you think you have ever gone through a period, no matter how short or long, in which you felt you were suffering? (Probe for resolution)

RELIGIOUS/SPIRITUAL BELIEFS ANDLIFE PRINCIPLES

We are just about finished. I just have some final questions that have more of a philosophical tone.

Do you think that there is a difference between a religious person and a spiritual person?

How would you describe yourself?

You told me that you are a ____________________ (religion).

Can you tell me the importance of your religious/spiritual beliefs in your life?

How does your faith help you in your day to day life as a caregiver?
(Probe for how, why)

Do you believe in an afterlife? If yes, **what do you think it will be like?**

What is the major principle you live by?

When you look in the mirror, what do you see?(If this is answered with a joke, ask:

When you look inside yourself, what do you see?

What are your goals right now?

When you wake up in the morning, what is the first thing you think about?

What makes you happy right now?

Can you name one or two of your major accomplishments in life?

Is there anything you wish I would have asked you and didn't,
Or is there something you would like to tell me in relation to our conversation today?

REFERENCES

Abrams, D. (1992). Processes of Social Identification. In Glynis M. Breakwell (Ed.), *Social Psychology of Identity and the Self-Concept* (pp. 55–99). London: Surry University Press.

Adler, M. (2012). Collective identity formation and collective action framing in a Mexican "movement of movements" *InterfaAU: A Journal for and about Social Movements, 4*(1), 287–315.

Adler, R., & Mehta, R. (2014). *Catalyzing technology to support family caregiving IV*. Bethesda, MD: National Alliance of Caregiving.

Aldwin, C., & Gilmer, D. (2013). *Health, illness, and optimal aging: Biological and psychosocial perspectives*. New York, NY: Springer.

American Civil Rights Union. (2014). *The truth about Jim Crow*. Alexandria, VA: ACRU Publications.

American History Archives. (2015). Military resources: Korean War. Washington, DC.

Anderson, J., & Turner, W. (2010). When caregivers are in need of care: African-American caregivers' preferences for their own later life care. *Journal of Aging Studies, 24*(1), 65–73.

Appy, C. G. (1993). *Working-class war: American combat soldiers and Vietnam*. Chapel Hill, NC: University of North Carolina Press.

Archbold, P. (1983). Impact of parent-caring on women. *Family Relations, 32*(1), 39–45.

Baldor, L. (2008). Black military officers rare 60 years after military desegregated. *The Huffington Post*, July 23, as cited in Black, H. K. (2015). Three generations: Three Wars. *The Gerontologist 56*(1), 33–41. doi: 10.1093/geron/gnv122.

Baldwin, J. (1961). *The last interview*. Interview by Studs Terkel. Brooklyn, NY: Melville Press.

Beaver County Times. (1973). Philadelphia General Hospital Closes. Beaver County, PA.

Becker, G. (1997). *Disrupted lives*. Berkeley, CA: University of California Press.

Beidler, P. D. (2004). *Late thoughts on an old war: The legacy of Vietnam*. Athens, GA: University of Georgia Press.

Bellah, R. N., Madsen, R., Sullivan, W. M., Swidler, A., & Tipton, S. M. (1985). *Habits of the heart: Individualism and commitment in American life*. Berkeley: University of California Press.

Black, H. K. (2001). Jake's story: A middle aged, working class man's physical and spiritual journey toward death. *Qualitative Health Research, 11*(3), 293–307.

Black, H. K. (2006). *Soul pain: The meaning of suffering in later life*. Amityville, NY: Baywood Press.

Black, H. K. (2010). The person in Alzheimer's disease. In L. Bregman (Ed). *Religion, death, and dying: Perspectives on dying and death* (pp. 52–70). Santa Barbara, CA: Praeger.

Black, H. K. (2011). The influence of African-American elders' belief systems on health interactions. *Journal of Religion and Spirituality in Social Work: Social Thought, 31*(3), 81–97.

Black, H. K. (2016). Three generations; three wars: African-American veterans. *The Gerontologist, 56*(1), 55–99.

Black, H. K., Caruso, C., Santanello, H., & Rubinstein, R. (2014). Managing threats against autonomy in old age. *Nursing Research, 62*(6), 430–437. doi: 10.1097/NNR.0000000000000003.

Black, H. K., Groce, J. T., & Harmon, C. (2011). *From zero to eighty: Narratives of racism, suffering, survival, and transformation*. Bloomington, IN: IUniverse.

Black, H. K., Hannum, S., Rubinstein, R. L., & DeMedeiros, K. (2015). Generativity in elderly African-American Oblate Sisters of Providence. *The Gerontologist, 56*(3), 559–568. doi: 10.1093/geront/gnu091.

Black, H. K., & Rubinstein, R. L. (2000). *Old souls: Aged women, poverty and the experience of God*. New York, NY: Aldine de Gruyter.

Black, H. K., & Rubinstein, R. L. (2004). Themes of suffering in later life. *Journal of Gerontology, Social Sciences, 59*(1), S17–S24.

Black, H. K., & Santanello, H. (2012). The salience of family worldview in mourning an elderly husband and father. *The Gerontologist, 52*(4), 472–483. doi: 10.1093/geront/gnr148.

Black, H. K., Schwartz, A., Caruso, C., & Hannum, S. (2008). How personal control mediates suffering: Elderly husbands' narratives of caregiving. *Journal of Men's Studies, 16*(2), 177–192.

Black, H. K., & Thompson, W. H. (2012). A war within a war: A World War II Buffalo soldier's story. *Journal of Men's Studies, 20*(1), 8–17.

Bowers, W. T., Hammond, W. M., & MacGarrigle, G. L. (1996). *Black soldier white army: The 24th Infantry Regiment*. Center of Military History, United States Army. Washington, DC.

Brandstadter, J., & Greave, W. (1994). The aging self: Stabilizing and protective processes. *Developmental Review, 14*, 52–80.

Bregman, L. (2014). *The ecology of spirituality*. Waco, TX: Baylor University Press. Press.

Brodaty, H., & Donkin, M. (2009). Family caregivers of people with dementia. *Dialogues in Clinical Neuroscience, 11*(2), 217–228.

Brummet, B., & Dilworth-Anderson, P. (2012). Associations of social support and 8-year follow up depressive symptoms: Differences in African American and white caregivers. *Clinical Gerontologist, 35*(4), 289–302.

Calasanti, T., & King, N. (2007). Taking "women's work" like a man: Husbands' experiences of care work. *The Gerontologist, 47*(4), 516–527.

Cassel, E. (1982). *The nature of suffering and the goals of medicine*. New York, NY: Oxford University Press.

Chapman, G. C. Jr. (1979). Black theology and theology of hope. In G. S. Wilmore & J. H. Cone (Eds.), *African American religious studies: An interdisciplinary anthology* (pp. 193–217). Durham, NC: Duke University Press.

Charmaz, K. (1999). Stories of suffering: Subjective tales and research narratives. *Qualitative Health Research, 9*, 362–382.

Chisholm, L., Weech-Maldonado, R., Laberge, A., Feng-Chang Lin, & Hyer, K. (2013). Nursing home quality and financial performance: Does the racial composition of residents matter? *Health Services Research*, *48*(6), 2060–2080. doi: 10.1111/1475-6773.12079

Climo, J., & Cattell, M. (2002). *Social memory and history: Anthropological perspectives*. Walnut Creek, CA: AltaMira Press.

Colby, S., & Ortman, J. (2015). *Projections of the size and composition of the U.S. population: 2014 to 2060*, Current Population Reports, P25–1143. Washington, DC: US Census Bureau.

Cone, J. (1970). *A Black theology of liberation*. Philadelphia, PA: Lippincott.

Cone, J. (1979). *African American religious studies: An interdisciplinary anthology*. G. S. Wilmore & J. H. Cone (Eds.). Durham, NC: Duke University Press.

Courtenay, W. (2000). Constructions of masculinity and their influence on men's well-being: A theory of gender and health. *Social Science & Medicine*, *50*, 1385–1401.

Daniel, J., Deering, M. J., & Murray, M. (2014). Using health IT to put the person at the center of their health and care by 2020. Issue Brief, Office of the National Coordinator, Health Information Technology, pp. 3–8, Washington, DC.

Dassel, K. B., & Carr, D. C. (2016). Does dementia caregiving accelerate frailty? Findings from the health and retirement study. *Gerontologist*, *56*, 444–450.

David, E. J. R. (2013). *Internalized oppression: The psychology of marginalized groups*. York, NY: Springer.

Dees, M., with Fiffer, S. (1991). *A season for justice*. New York, NY MacMillan.

Desjarlais, R., & Throop, E. (1997). Phenomenological approaches in anthropology. *Annual Review of Anthropology*, *40*, 87–102.

Dilworth-Anderson, P., Goodwin, P., & Williams, S. (2004). Can culture help explain the physical health effects of caregiving over time among African American caregivers? *Journal of Gerontology*, *59*(3), S138–S145.

Du Bois, W. E. B. (1903a). *The Negro church in America*. Atlanta, GA: Atlanta University Press.

Du Bois, W. E. B. (1903b). *The souls of black folk*. New York, NY: Pocket Books.

Eisenhandler, S. (2003). *Keeping the faith in late life*. New York, NY: Springer.

Erikson, E. H. (1963). *Childhood and society*. New York, NY: W.W. Norton.

Erikson, E., Erikson, J., & Kivnick, H. (1986). *Vital Involvement in Old Age*. New York: W.W. Norton and Co.

Fiske, A., Wetherell, J., & Gatz, M. (2009). Depression in older adults. *Annual Review of Clinical Psychology*, *5*, 363–389. doi: 10.1146/annurev.clinpsy.032408.153621

Flyvbjerg, B. (2006). Five misunderstandings about case study research. *Qualitative Inquiry*, *12*(2), 219–245.

Frazier, E. F. (1974).*The Negro Church in America*. New York, NY Schocken.

Freedman, V. A., Corman, J. C., & Carr, D. (2014). Is spousal caregiving associated with enhanced well-being? New evidence from the panel study of income dynamics. *Journals of Gerontology, Series B*, *69*(6), 861–869. doi: 10.1093/geronb/gbu004

Gadamer, H. G. (1975). Hermeneutics and social science. *Philosophy Social Criticism/ Cultural Hermeneutics*, *2*(4), 307–316.

Gallagher, B. (2014). The Vietnam War and the Civil Rights movement. *American Studies Resources Centre, Aldham Robarts Library, John Moores University*. American Studies Today Online. Liverpool, UK. Posted 20 February 2014.

Gaugler, J. E., Reese, M., & Mittelman, M. S. (2016). Effects of the Minnesota adaptation of the NYU caregiver intervention on depressive symptoms and quality of life for adult child caregivers of persons with dementia. *American Journal of Geriatric Psychiatry*, *23*(11), 1179–1192. doi: 10.1016/j.jagp.2015.06.007.

Geertz, C. (1973). *The interpretation of cultures*. New York, NY: Springer.

Gelder, K. (2007). *Subcultures: Cultural histories and social practice*. New York, NY: Routledge.

Given, B., Sherwood, P. R., Given, C. W. (2008). What knowledge and skills do caregivers need? *American Journal of nursing, 9*(108), 28–34. doi: 10.1097/01.NAJ 0000336408.52872.d2.

Groce, J. (2002). *Caregivers: For better or worse*. Workshop held at Widener University. October 10. Chester, PA.

Gutierrez, G. (1988). *A theology of liberation. Revised edition*. Maryknoll, NY: Orbis Books.

HSC Foundation. (2010). *The overlooked caregiver: A series of listening sessions*. National Caucus and Center on Black Aged, Inc. Washington, DC: HSC Publications.

Hamilton, J. B., & Sandelowski, M. (2004). Types of social support in African Americans with cancer. *Oncology Nursing Forum, 31*, 792–800.

Hanlon, N. (2012). *Masculinities, care and equality: Identity and nurture in men's lives*. Basingstoke, Hampshire, UK: Palgrave MacMillan.

Hasselkus, B., & Murray, B. (2007). Everyday occupation, well-being, and identity: The experience of caregivers in families with dementia. *The American Journal of Occupational Therapy, 61*(1), 9–20.

Healthcare System Foundation. (2007). *Male caregiving: Creating a research, programmatic, and policy agenda for an emerging public health issue*. College Park, MD.

Hines, P. M., & Boyd-Franklin, N. (1996). African American families. In M. McGoldrick, J. Giordano, & P. J. K. Pearce (Eds), *Ethnicity and family therapy* (2nd ed., pp. 66–84). New York, NY: Guilford Press.

Hopp, F., & Thomas, S. (2014). Go to the hospital or stay at home? A qualitative study of expected hospital decision making among older African Americans with advanced heart failure. *Journal of Gerontological Social Work, 57*(1), 4–23.

Horowitz, M. (2012). Self-identity theory and research methods. *Journal of Research Practice, 8*(2), 12–18.

HSC Foundation. (2010). *The overlooked caregiver: A series of listening sessions*. National Caucus and Center on Black Aged, Inc. Washington, DC: HSC Publications.

Husserl, E. (1964). *The idea of phenomenology* (trans W. P. Alston & G. Nakhnikian). The Hague, the Netherlands: Nijhoff. (Original work published 1907)

Jacobs, E. A., Rolle, I., Ferrans, C. E., Whitaker, E. E., & Warnecke, R. B. (2006). Understanding African Americans' views of the trustworthiness of physicians. *Journal of General Internal Medicine, 21*(6), 642–647. doi: 10.1111/j.1525-1497.2006.00485.x

Janevic, M. R., & Connell, C. M. (2001). Racial, ethnic, and cultural differences in the dementia caregiving experience: *The Gerontologist, 41*(3), 334–347. doi: 10.1093/geront/41.3.334

Janoff-Bulman, R., & Carnes, N. C. (2013). Surveying the moral landscape: Moral motives and group-based moralities. *Personality and Social Psychology Review, 17*, 242–247

Kaufman, A., & Tang, M. (2010). Social support, caregiver burden, and life satisfaction in a sample of rural African American and white caregivers of older persons with dementia. *Journal of Gerontological Social Work, 53*(3), 251–269.

Kelly, K., Reinhard, S., & Brooks-Danso, A. (2008). Executive summary: Professional partners supporting family caregivers. *American Journal of Nursing, 108*(9), 6–12.

Kidron, C. A. (2003). Surviving a distant past: A case study of the cultural construction of trauma descendant identity. *Ethos, 31*(4), 513–544.

Kim, S., & Ferraro, K. (2014). Do productive activities reduce inflammation in later life? *The Gerontologist*, *54*(5), 830–839.

Kitwood, T. (1997). *Dementia reconsidered: The person comes first*. Buckingham, UK: Open University Press.

Kleinman, A. (1980). *Patients and healers in the context of culture: An exploration of the borderland between anthropology, medicine, and psychiatry*. Berkeley, CA: University of California Press.

Koltko-Rivera, M. E. (2004). The psychology of worldviews. *Review of General Psychology*, *8*(1), 3–58. doi: 10.1037/1089-2680.8.1.3

Kotre, J. (2005). Generativity: Reshaping the past into the future. *Science & Theology News*, September, 42–43.

Kramer, B. (2005). Men caregivers: An overview. In *Men as caregivers* pp 3–19. Amherst, NY: Prometheus Books.

Kramer, B., & Thompson, E. (2005). *Men as caregivers*. Amherst, NY: Prometheus Books.

Lane, G., & King, D. (2012). "The hidden caregiver": Kinship caregivers and lessons learned from dementia family caregiving. *Clinical Gerontologist*, *35*(2), 195–203.

Lane, R. (1991). *William Dorsey's Philadelphia and ours: On the past and future of the black city in America*. New York, NY: Oxford University Press.

Levine, C. (2008). Needed: Nursing and social work leadership. *American Journal of Nursing*, *108*(9), 13–15.

Lin, I. F., Fee, H. R., & Wu, H. S. (2012). Negative and positive caregiving experiences: A closer look at the intersection of gender and relationships. *Family Relations*, *61*, 343–358. doi:10.1111/j.1741-3729.2011.00692.x

Lincoln, C., & Mamiya, L. H. (1990). *The Black Church in the African American experience*. Durham, NC: Duke University Press.

Lipsyte, R. (1988). An outsider joins the team. *New York Times Magazine*, May 22.

Lotterhos, F. H. (2015). *Men cry: Embodiments of masculinity in Western cinema circa 1999*. Undergraduate honors thesis. Paper 814. University of Colorado, Boulder.

Luborsky, M. (1993). The identification and analyses of themes and patterns. In J. Gubrium & A. Sankar (Eds)., *Qualitative methods in aging research* (pp. 189–210). Thousand Oaks, CA: Sage.

Luborsky, M., & Rubinstein, R. (1995). Sampling in qualitative research: Rationale, issues, and methods. *Research on Aging*, *17*(1), 79–113.

Mace, N., & Rabine, P. (1981). *The 36 hour day: A family guide to caring for persons with Alzheimer's disease, related dementing illnesses, and memory loss in later life* (1st ed.). Baltimore, MD: Johns Hopkins University Press.

Mack, K. (2005). *A decade of informal caregiving*. Washington, DC: Center on an Aging Society, Georgetown University.

Martin, E. (1987). *The woman in the body*. Boston, MA: Beacon Press.

Mattis, J. S., & Jaggers, R. J. (2001). A relational framework for the study of religiosity and spirituality in the lives of African Americans. *Journal of Community Psychology*, *29*, 519–530.

Mattis, J. S., Murray, Y. F., Hatcher, C. A., Hearn, K. D., Lawhon, G. D., Murphy, E. J., . . . Washington, T. A. (2001). Religiosity, spirituality, and the subjective quality of African American men's friendships: An exploratory study. *Journal of Adult Development*, *8*(4), 221–230. doi:10.1023/A:1011338511989

McAdams, D. P. (2012). Exploring psychological themes through life-narrative accounts. In J. A. Holstein & J. F. Gubrium (Eds.), *Varieties of narrative analysis* (pp. 15–32). Thousand Oaks, CA. Sage.

Mead, G. H. (1932). *The philosophy of the present*. New York, NY: Prometheus Books.

Mead, G. H. (1934). *Mind, self, and society*. Edited by Charles W. Morris. Chicago, IL: University of Chicago Press.

Micka, K. (2006). *Men as caregivers: Beyond toughing it out*. Article 6, Citrus Heights, CA: Deloro Caregiver Resource Center.

Minton, R. (1951). The history of Mercy-Douglass Hospital. *Journal of the National Medical Association, 43*(3), 153.

Mischler, E. (1986). *Research interviewing: Context and narrative*. Cambridge, MA: Harvard University Press.

Moore, J. (2010). *Caregiving: An exploration of African-American male caregiver roles in Texas*. Masters/Doctoral dissertation, University of Texas.

Morano, C., & King, M. (2010). Lessons learned from implementing a psycho-educational intervention for African American dementia caregivers. *Dementia, 9*(4), 558–568.

Morling, B., & Evered, S. (2006). Secondary control reviewed and defined. *Psychological Bulletin, 132*, 269–296.

Murphy, R. (1987). *The body silent*. New York, NY: W.W. Norton.

Mutua, A. D. (2006). *Progressive black masculinities*. New York, NY: Routledge.

National Alliance for Caregiving (NAC) and the American Association of Retired Persons (AARP). (2015). *Caregiving in the US*. Bethesda, MD: Author.

PBS Television, WHYY Channel 12. (2015). *American Experience. Freedom Riders*. Philadelphia, PA.

PBS Television, WHYY Channel 12. (2014). *The Sixties*. Philadelphia, PA.

Peveto, C., & Hayslip, B. (2004). *Cultural changes in attitudes toward death, dying, and bereavement*. New York, NY: Springer.

Pharr, J., Francis, C., Terry, C., & Clark, M. (2014). Culture, caregiving, and health: Exploring the influence of culture on family caregiver experiences. *ISRN Public Health Volume 2014* (2014), Article ID689826, 8 pages http://dx.doi.org/10.1155/2014/689826

Phillipson, C., & Biggs, S. (1998). Modernity and identity: Themes and perspectives in the study of older adults. *Journal of Aging and Identity, 3*(1), 11–23.

Pierre, M., Mahalik, J., & Woodland, M. (2001). The effects of racism, African self consciousness and psychological functioning on black masculinity: A historical and social adaptation framework. *Journal of African-American Men, 6*(2), 19–39.

Pinquart, M., & Sorensen, S. (2005). Ethnic differences in stressors, resources, and psychological outcomes of family caregiving: A meta-analysis. *Gerontologist, 45*(1), 90–106.

Raboteau, A. (1978). *Slave religion: The invisible institution in the antebellum South*. New York, NY: Oxford University Press.

Radley, A., & Billig, M. (1996). Accounts of health and illness: Dilemmas and representations. *Sociology of Health and Illness, 18*(Issue 2), 220–240.

Reinhard, S., Brooks-Danso, A.,. Kelly, K., & Mason, D. (2008). How are you doing? *American Journal of Nursing, 108*(9 Suppl), 4–5. doi: 10.1097/01.NAJ.0000336398.91882.

Reissman, C. (1993). *Narrative analysis*. Newbury Park, CA: Sage.

Rexroth, D., & Friedland, R. (2010). Lessons learned regarding recruitment to the National African American Alzheimer Disease Health Literacy Program. *Alzheimer Disease and Associated Disorders, 24* (Supplement), 54–57.

Ribeiro, O., Paul, C., & Nogueira, C. (2007). Real men, real husbands: Caregiving and masculinities in later life. *Journal of Aging Studies, 21*(4), 302–313.

Rosenbaum, S. (2015). Clash of the Titans: Medicaid Meets Private Health Insurance. *Yale Journal of Health Policy, Law, and Ethics*: *15*(1), Article 11. Available at: http://digitalcommons.law.yale.edu/yjhple/vol15/iss1/11

Rubinstein, R. (1992). Anthropological methods in gerontological research: Entering the world of meaning. *Journal of Aging Studies*, *6*, 57–66.

Rubinstein, R. L., Girling, L., de Medeiros, K., Brazda, M., & Hannum, S. (2014). Extending the framework of generativity theory through research: A qualitative study. *The Gerontologist*. Advance online publication. doi: 10.1093/geront/gnu009

Russell, R. (2007). The work of elderly men caregivers: From public careers to an unseen world. *Men and Masculinities*, *9*(31), 298–314.

Sampson, C. A. (2015). Hymn lining: A black church tradition with roots in Europe. *The Spectrum: A Scholars Day Journal*, *3*, Article 9. Available at http://digitalcommons.brockport.edu/spectrum/vol3/iss1/9.

Scharlach, A. (2008). Historical overview. *Journal of Nursing*, *108*(9), 16–22.

Schroots, J., & Birren, J. (2002). The study of lives in progress: Approaches to research on life stories. In G. D. Rowles & N. E. Schoenberg (Eds.), *Qualitative gerontology: A contemporary perspective* (pp. 51–65). New York, NY Springer.

Shanas, E., & Streib, G. (1965). *Social structure and the family: Generational relations*. Englewood Cliffs, NJ: Prentice-Hall.

Shear, M. K. (2012). Grief and mourning gone awry: Pathway and course of complicated grief. *Dialogues in Clinical Neuroscience, 14*(2), 119–128.

Silverman, D. (2001). *Interpreting qualitative data: Methods for analyzing talk, text, and interaction*. Thousand Oaks, CA: Sage.

Skinner, E. (1996). A guide to constructs of control. *Journal of Personality and Social Psychology*, *71*(3), 549–570.

Sneed, J. R., & Whitbourne, S. K. (2003). Identity processing and self-consciousness in middle and later adulthood. *Journal of Gerontology B Psychological Sciences and Social Sciences*, *58*(6), 313–319.

Snellman, I., Gustafsson, C., &Gustafsson, L. (2012). Patients' and caregivers' attributes in a meaningful care encounter: Similarities and notable differences. *ISRN Nursing*, Article ID 320145, doi.org/10.5402/2012/320145.

Solorzano, M., Ceja, M., Yosso, T. (2000). Critical race theory, racial microaggressions, and campus racial climate: The experiences of African American college students. *The Journal of Negro Education*, *69*, No. 1/2, Knocking at Freedom's Door: Race, Equity, and Affirmative Action in U.S. Higher Education. (Winter - Spring, 2000), pp. 60–73.

Stewart, P. (2008). Care provision for African American elders: Family attitudes and strategies. *Journal of Intergenerational Relationships*, *6*(1), 61–81.

Stouffer, S. (1949). *The American soldier: Adjustment during army life*. Princeton, NJ: Princeton University Press.

Strauss, A., & Corbin, J. (1990). Basics of qualitative research. Thousand Oaks, CA: Sage Publications.

Thomas, N., Groce, J., & Cooper, R. (2003). Changing direction: Rites of passage programs for African-American older men. *Journal of African-American Studies,* 7(3), 3–14.

Thompson, E. (2005). What's unique about men's caregiving. In *Men as caregivers* (pp. 20–47). Amherst, NY: Prometheus Books.

Tise, Olivia T. (2015). The support group experience of older male caregivers in providing care for a relative with dementia. Master of Social Work Clinical Research Papers. Paper 534. http://sophia.stkate.edu/msw_papers/534

Troll, L. (1971). The family of later life: A decade review. *Journal of Marriage and the Family, 33*(2), 263–290.

Tumulty, K. (2014). The Great Society at 50. May 17, *The Washington Post*.

US Census Bureau. (2015). *Population projections of the United States by age, sex, race, and Hispanic origin: 1993–2050*. Current Population Reports, P25–1104.

US Department of Health and Human Services. (2011). *A profile of older Americans: 2011*. Administration on Aging.

Van Manen, M. (1990). *Researching lived experience*. Ontario, Canada: University of Western Ontario.

Vitaliano, P. P., Zhang, J., & Scanlan, J. M. (2003). Is caregiving hazardous to your health? A meta-analysis. *Psychological Bulletin, 129*(6), 946–972.

Volicer, L., & van der Steen, J. (2014). Outcome measures for dementia in the advanced stage and at the end of life. *Advances in Geriatrics*, Article ID 346485, http://dx.doi.org/10.1155/2014/346485

Weinland, J. (2009). The lived experience of African American male caregivers. *American Journal of Men's Health, 3*(1), 6–24.

Williams, R. (2001). Department of Defense salutes African-American Korean War veterans. *Department of Defense News*, 7, 2.

Wilmore, G. (1989). *African American religious studies: An interdisciplinary anthology*. G. S. Wilmore & J. H. Cone (Eds.). General Introduction, 1–12. Durham, NC: Duke University Press.

Wilmore, G. S. (1983). *Black religion and Black radicalism*. Maryknoll, NY: Orbis.

Wing Sue, D. (2010). *Microaggressions in everyday life: Race, gender, and sexual orientation*. New York, NY: Wiley.

Wong, C., & Wallhagen, M. (2014). Family caregivers of individuals with frontotemporal dementia: Examining the relationship between coping and caregiver physical and mental health. *Journal of Gerontological Nursing, 40*(1), 30–40.

Yang, S. Y. (2008). Real-life contextual manifestation of wisdom. *International Journal of Aging and Human Development, 67*(4), 273–303.

INDEX